Yoga

PURE AND SIMPLE

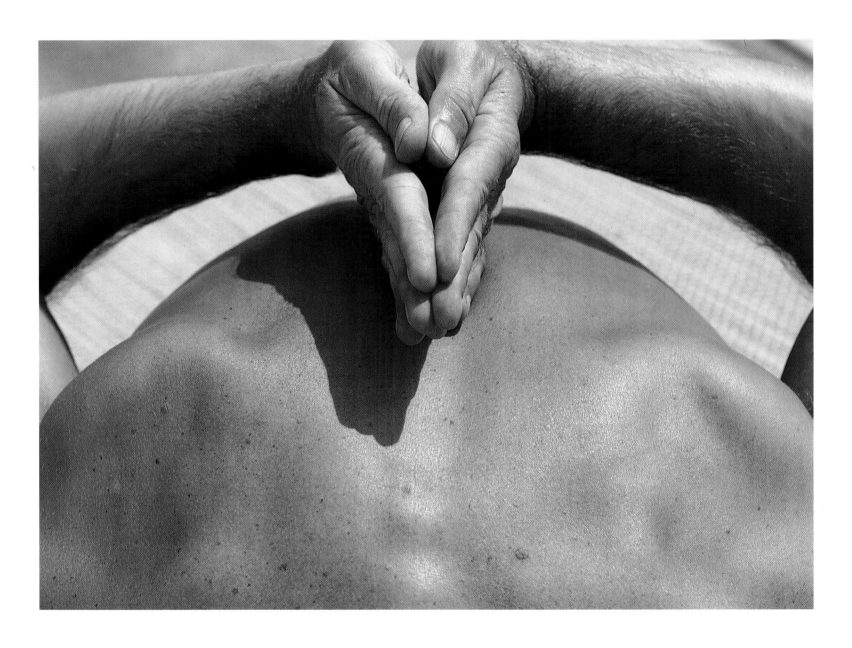

Yoga

PURE AND SIMPLE

Kisen

HAY
HOUSE

Carlsbad, California • Sydney, Australia

To Celia and Eddie, my mum and dad, who have only ever given and wanted nothing in return

Other Hay House Titles of Related Interest

Books

BodyChange™: *The 21-Day Fitness Program for Changing Your Body . . . and Changing Your Life,* by Montel Williams and Wini Linguvic

The Body Knows: *How to Tune In to Your Body and Improve Your Health,* by Caroline Sutherland, Medical Intuitive

Eating in the Light: *Making the Switch to Vegetarianism on Your Spiritual Path,* by Doreen Virtue, Ph.D., and Becky Prelitz, M.F.T., R.D.

Heal Your Body A-Z, by Louise L. Hay

Ultimate Pilates: *Achieve the Perfect Body Shape,* by Dreas Reyneke (available ??)

Audio Programs

How to Relax, by Carl Simonton, M.D.

Reversing Heart Disease, by Julian Whitaker, M.D.

Vital Energy: *The 7 Keys to Invigorate Body, Mind & Soul,* by David Simon, M.D.

Your Diet, Your Health, by Christiane Northrup, M.D.

The Zone: *Enter the Zone . . . the Diet That's Sweeping the Country,* by Barry Sears, Ph. D.

All of the above are available at your local bookstore, or may be ordered through Hay House, Inc.:

(800) 654-5126 or **(760) 431-7695**
(800) 650-5115 (fax) or **(760) 431-6948 (fax)**
www.hayhouse.com

© 2002 by Kisen

Published and distributed in the United States by: Hay House, Inc., P.O. Box 5100, Carlsbad, CA 92018-5100 • (800) 654-5126 • (800) 650-5115 (fax) • www.hayhouse.com
Hay House Australia Pty Ltd, P.O. Box 515, Brighton-Le-Sands NSW 2216 1800 023 516
e-mail: info@hayhouse.com.au

Editorial supervision: Jill Kramer • *Design:* Helen Lewis • *Interior photos:* Graham Atkins-Hughes

Cataloging-in-Publication Data available from the Library of Congress

ISBN 1-56170-985-9

05 04 03 02 4 3 2 1
1st printing, February 2002

Printed in France

Contents

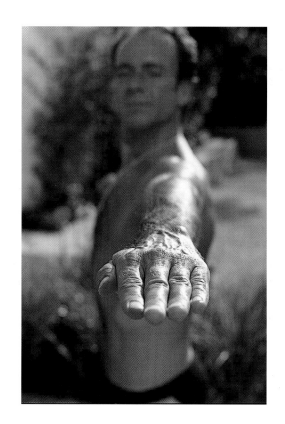

Preface

This book is essentially a manual of instruction and, as such, is rooted in the tangible realms of the how, the why, and the what happens when. It was born out of the repeated requests of students wishing to know how to structure their own practice. Although a good teacher is essential, particularly in the beginning, self-practice is where we really begin to develop.

The structure of the book is sequential; groups of postures are linked together to explain their relationship to each other, their purpose, and to promote fluency within structure. These postures and sequences have proved to be most effective for the widest range of students. They are designed to challenge, educate, and encourage students of all ages and physical types, and provide a firm foundation from which self-practice can develop safely and effectively.

It is best to read through the introductions to each chapter first, and to get a feel of the sequences before undertaking any practice, as this will establish an understanding of the principles and pertinence of practice from the outset. Few references are given to the esoteric and mystical aspects of practice, as I wanted the information to be clear, concise, and practical. All of the mysterious and magical elements afforded by regular practice are therefore yours to discover as practice and intimacy deepen.

Kisen

Introduction

The word *yoga* is commonly translated as "union," to unite or to bind. Personally I prefer to define yoga as "to reunite, to restore, and to bring together," as the practice of yoga is a process of disentanglement and reconnection. It is not so much a matter of learning something new to us; it is more a matter of unlearning. We must locate, identify, and break the bonds of the habitual patterns of action we have made, which have robbed us of our natural grace and poise. Our various postural imbalances reveal areas of tension, immobility, and resistance. The physical tensions we carry in the body are the results of both the circumstances we have met throughout our lives and our reaction to them. They are, therefore, largely the product of mind and are both the source and result of our dissatisfaction. Undoing the wrongs we have done to our bodies is also the responsibility of mind, and it is by the direct, conscious application of mind to this task that the one benefits the other. The medium used to direct the flow of the conscious mind through the body is the breath—our spirit. The three elements that constitute life—body, spirit, and mind—are all thus treated equally and with increasing intimacy. This is the practice that we call yoga.

Using this book
The sequences of this book are designed to deepen our intimate awareness of and connection with every aspect of our being.

This has very little to do with conventional understanding of fitness, although with regular practice you will become very fit. Nor has it particularly to do with flexibility or strength, though once again it will provide great strength and flexibility. It doesn't even have to do with relaxation, but it will make you truly relaxed. The great gift and power of this practice is that it returns what has become separate to a state of wholeness. Disorganization reveals weakness and confusion, whereas a combined force is powerful and effective.

The initial impact of practice seems to be placed firmly upon the body. However, the body must be guided by the mind and enlivened by the energy provided by the breath. Therefore, realize from the outset that the resistance experienced when practicing yoga is found in the mind muscle as well as the corporeal self, and that it is the dissolution of resistance that leads to harmony and liberation. See also the Guidelines for practice on page 17.

The art of good practice
At first, the practice of the postures can be seen as trying to tame a wild stallion. The body is unruly and rebellious, and will not readily submit to the instructions and wishes of the mind. The mind may find the stubbornness and strength of the body hard to hold and control inner vigilance. Indeed, composure and awareness need to be harnessed with pure energy if the body is

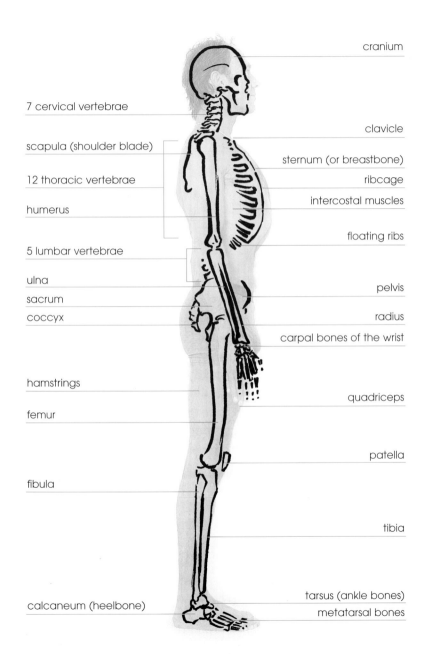

cranium

7 cervical vertebrae

clavicle

scapula (shoulder blade)

sternum (or breastbone)

12 thoracic vertebrae

ribcage

intercostal muscles

humerus

floating ribs

5 lumbar vertebrae

ulna

pelvis

sacrum

coccyx

radius

carpal bones of the wrist

hamstrings

quadriceps

femur

patella

fibula

tibia

tarsus (ankle bones)

calcaneum (heelbone)

metatarsal bones

Although a deep knowledge of anatomy is not essential for practice, a certain basic understanding is useful, as throughout the book, reference is made to various bones, joints, organs, and muscle groups. The diagram on the left and the photograph on page 12 illustrate all of the parts of the body mentioned in the text.

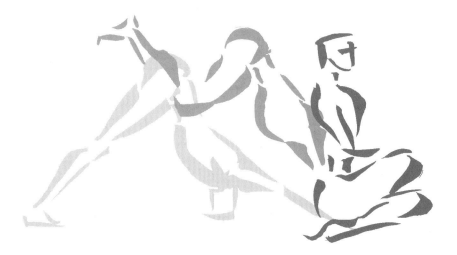

There is a great inherent power that comes from synchronizing the breath with movement. By paying careful attention to the flow of the breath, movements become graceful and breathing capacity is increased. Jumping forward on an in-breath from Dog Pose to a sitting position has the effect of activating and locking the lower abdominal muscles, while at the same time opening and expanding the lungs and ribs. In the process, the diaphragm regains its elasticity, and the abdominal muscles become firm and strong.

to be encouraged to comply and for the mind to cease to struggle. Our breath is the source of this energy and, indeed, of all life. The sequences and techniques described have the effect of increasing not only our ability to deliver and control this energy, but also to increase our awareness of the influence of the breath upon the body/mind.

With the awareness of breath comes an understanding of the nature of physical, emotional, and psychological conditioning. It is only by developing this awareness that the dual bonds of attachment and resistance can be broken. The practice of these forms, therefore, is a process of deepening awareness and intimacy of ourselves multidimensionally. Our weaknesses, imbalances, and hidden tensions are all brought under the microscope of awareness for inspection. The result of this close attention is that our tensions dissolve and the innate intelligence of the body is reawakened—multifaceted integration is thus developed.

The sequences and techniques described in this book are the instruments that instruct us in the art of awareness. They are precise, practical, and have a holistic effect. Structured in rhythm and fluency, they reveal the many dimensions of experience that help us to move from sensation, to information, to knowledge, to practical wisdom. It is from our personal involvement with these forms that we begin to uncover our latent strength and awareness of ourselves as evolving beings and open the door to our true potential.

Learning to breathe

There is a basic universal law that proclaims that whatever is nourished grows and flourishes; whatever is ignored decays and dies. Undertaking the study and practice of these forms provides nourishment, as they force us to take responsibility for ourselves in a mature and sensitive manner that reflects how we are in this world. Our essential nourishment is derived and dependent upon our ability to breathe.

A special breathing technique is used throughout each sequence to glean the most energy we can from the air we breathe. The postures and movements between postures are used both to educate and challenge the flow of this special breath. The body/mind is thereby stimulated, enlivened, and refreshed, and inner order is reestablished. The technique we employ is called Ujjayi breathing, which means upward surge of power. The true meaning of the word *inspiration* reveals the same quality. This technique has a tremendously powerful effect upon the entire bio-energy systems of the body.

- It encourages and promotes a deep absorption of vital energy into the bloodstream.
- The quality, richness, and chemical composition of the blood directly influences all of the tissues, fluids, and nerve impulses of the body.
- This increases the vitality and enhances the condition of the whole organism.
- In turn, this provides an elevated capacity for living.

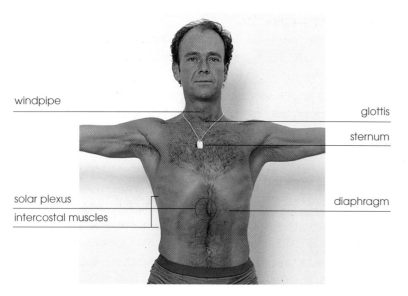

windpipe

glottis

sternum

solar plexus

intercostal muscles

diaphragm

The technique of Ujjayi breathing

The basic technique is quite simple; all you need to do is to exert a little internal pressure, or grip, upon the root of the throat at the point of the glottis. This applied force produces two immediate and distinct effects.

1 The breath becomes resonant and audible. The in-breath is warm and fragrant and produces a sibilant sound Saah; the out-breath is cool, lacks fragrance, and makes an aspirate sound Haam. These two sounds are the result of the broadening of the windpipe, which is manufactured by the slight lock placed on the glottis and not by adding any humming or snoring sounds. The resonance is the result of the vibration made by the passage of the breath through the windpipe. Any additional sounds are an indication that the technique is not quite right. It is therefore essential that an understanding of this subtle action and resultant sound is established from the outset.

2 The breath becomes deeper and longer. It is quite remarkable that simply by the application of this action, suddenly and with very little effort we dramatically increase our ability to breathe freely and deeply.

A description of how to breathe effectively is given opposite. It is important that you read this, as breathing correctly is intrinsic to good yoga practice. The resonance and increase in the depth and length of each breath has a very profound effect upon the entirety of our practice. For if breath is life, it follows that the greater the influence and control we have over our breath, the greater the mastery we have of ourselves. The subtlety and delicacy of the sounds made by the passage of breath through the windpipe have two distinct benefits:

- The sounds aid in maintaining awareness, contact, and focus on the breath.
- The vibration itself has a direct and soothing effect upon the nervous system.

All vibration produces sound, and sound is a transformative vehicle. The use of mantras in some practices is an example of the power and use of sound to heighten and alter states of consciousness. In this system, our breath can be seen as the mantra of life.

Constant awareness on the tone of each breath establishes a cellular command communication that originates in the micro-motions that we call vibration. Intercellular communication through nerve tissue controls both the functioning of the body and also interprets, translates, and processes the information received through the senses from the external world to the inner. It does not take a neurologist to understand that regulating and improving the functioning of the nervous system is bound to mitigate the stresses and strains of life. By placing careful attention upon the refinement of the twin actions of depth and resonance, practice develops safely, naturally, and quickly.

Developing your practice

The questions posed by the various movements, postures, and sequences can only be successfully answered by the continuing refinement of this technique. In fact, the postures and movements between postures are physical conundrums designed specifically to instill the ability to manufacture smooth, deep, and resonant breath despite the impositions placed upon the respiratory system and our powers of concentration. The overt actions of the Sun exercises are therefore your starting point, as the principles of expansion and contraction are made implicit by the synchronization of sweeping movements, exactly with each breath. Give great care and attention to the actions, for these can all too easily challenge and disturb the smooth passage of the breath. It is by overcoming these difficulties that you will gain the greatest rewards.

The Sun exercises are the great educators of the respiratory system, but they also raise questions to encourage and further our understanding just as much as they explain and demonstrate the obvious. There are three significant problems posed by the Sun exercises to the breathing mechanism.

The purpose and refinement of all practice is to increase the intimacy and awareness that you have of your capacity to consciously direct energy into and throughout the body/mind. The range, diversity, and pertinence of every movement furthers our connection with, and control of, the vital force: our breath. Initially you will mainly be concerned with the obvious, immediate intensity of the sensations and the seeming complexity of the practice. However, as your awareness deepens, you will begin to see the simple within the complex and exchange resistance for indulgence. This transition only occurs through deliberate, precise, and sustained practice.

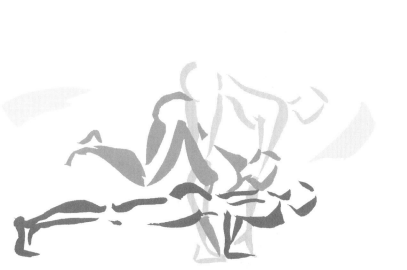

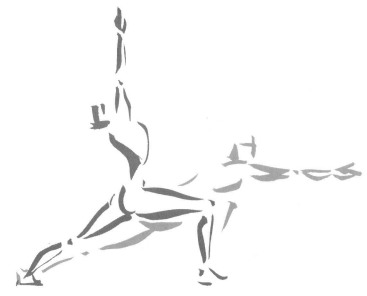

• The first question posed is the jump back to the floor, where the body is poised on the toes and hands. Exhaling smoothly and evenly throughout this movement compresses the lungs and ribcage and develops the intercostal muscles and abdominal wall. Any fluctuation in the sound of the breath during this and indeed every movement, indicates an area of immobility of an aspect of the lung, ribs, or spine. By repeated, sustained, and conscious practice of this action, the tidal flow of the breath is substantially increased. Tidal flow is the amount of breath we are able to exhale, it dictates the amount of stale carbon dioxide we can release from the body. More important, however, is the fact that the deeper we can exhale, the greater our capacity to inhale fresh vibrant energy. This is due to the elastic recoil of the lungs. which dictates our capacity to inhale.

• The most dramatic imposition placed upon the respiratory system by the Sun exercises is the movement from the Dog Pose (see page 25, right) to the elevation and lift into the standing posture. The challenge here is to step one leg forward and to lift the trunk and arms on a single, smooth inhalation. This simple action can seem very demanding if the ribs, spine, lungs, and abdomen are not working in harmony. Any hesitation, pause, or lack of smoothness is a direct indication of imbalance and/or rigidity. This sweeping, grand gesture is a powerful tool that promotes and breeds the ability to inhale and, in the process, to correct physical imbalance, exchanging the rigid for the flexible.

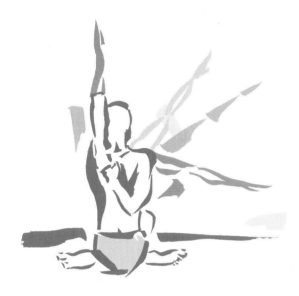

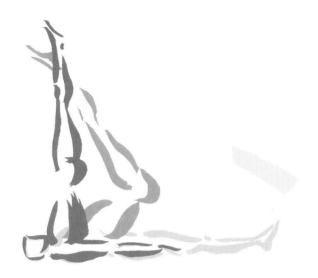

• The second movement of the first Sitting sequence (see page 66) describes the attitude and action necessary to gain full advantage of the resultant posture. Too often the information provided and established through the Sun and Standing sequences is ignored or neglected when we perform the Sitting, Inverted, and Supine sequences, as these sequences often use more refined actions. This is most evident in the reverse arm-lock. The arm running up the spine, bent back, must be extended up to its limit and kept long and firm as it is swept around the trunk to arrive high between the shoulder blades. The same is true of the upper arm, as concentrating upon these twin actions ensures that the chest is fully expanded and also educates the joints and muscles of the arms, shoulders, and back to their original form and thus restores natural poise and relieves tension.

• Although the Inverted postures are generally introspective and reflective, the first movement of the first sequence (see page 89) is akin to the vibrant, dramatic actions of the Sun sequences. The intelligence of this movement lies in the supportive action given by the arms and hands. The firm, bracing action of the arms directly influences the upper chest and back muscles. The demands made upon the respiratory system to simultaneously inhale and elevate the entire body smoothly and gracefully require diligence and deliver confidence. The basic principle of movement with and by each breath is most evident and important in this action.

Raising your levels of concentration

As practice develops, so will your acute awareness and understanding of the interrelationship of energy, body, and mind. Your levels of concentration will be heightened as you attend to the finer details. The gaze points are an example of the way in which the system of yoga targets and increases the powers of concentration and effects change through the subtlest of means.

Throughout the instructions given for each sequence, I detail specific points of the focus of the eyes. This helps you maintain conscious inner awareness and has a strong influence on the brain. Tension in the eyes contracts the brain and thus limits our potential awareness. Tightness or hardness of the eyes also indicates resistance. Conversely, concentrated visual attention, sustained by the muscles of the eyes, exercises a strong controlling power over wandering thoughts. By continually drawing attention to the softness and steadiness of the eyes, you will maintain an atmosphere of inner calm, which encourages the right attitude necessary for practice. Attending to each and every detail reveals the whole, and also depersonalizes the immediate intensity of some of the more obvious sensations. This is where your practice begins to mature and bear fruit.

However, it is important to realize as you begin your practice that you can only do what you, as an individual, can do. It is a dangerous mistake to adopt an image of how practice should be or what you should be able to do. But if the true value of your practice is to be translated into your way of being in this world, you must do as much as you can, engaging the whole of your being. Real value comes from the right attitude embodied in practical action. This is born out of the inner caliber of your heart/mind. It is not necessary to go to remote regions or the top of a mountain to find yourself. In this way, you only need to look inside to be enriched by the process of being alive. You can then practice, experience, incorporate, and express as a progressive individual who can admire the process and thereby enjoy yourself.

Guidelines for practice

In this book, I have provided you with a choice of sequences starting with the Sun exercises and then working through standing, sitting, inverted, and supine postures. The chapters on relaxation and meditation that follow describe the best way to end your practice session. The sequences and their order are designed so you can tailor your practice to as long or as short a time as you can manage. By taking one sequence from each chapter, you will work through a logical progression of postures, which will develop the physical aspect of being and educate and enliven the body/mind into the pertinence and power of practice. Follow these guidelines and pay careful attention to the instructions given for each posture and movement, and progress will be swift, safe, and satisfying.

- Sustained, regular practice is the key to success.
- Sporadic, occasional practice is virtually worthless.
- It is best to practice with an empty stomach. So first thing in the morning and early evening are the most beneficial times to begin practice.
- Wear as little as possible, or clothing that allows you to move freely, without restriction.
- Make sure that the area for practice is clean and tidy, as this establishes an orderly and simple quality of mind, which are the prerequisite elements necessary for effective practice.
- Always practice on a non-slip surface. A yoga mat is an ideal accessory, as not only does it provide adhesion and grip, but also simply by laying the mat out on the floor you have made the choice to begin. Too often you can talk yourself out of practice and into another cup of tea; setting out the mat establishes intention and provides impetus.
- Pay attention to the daily changes of your body/mind, and adjust your practice accordingly. Remember, we are all individuals and are dealing with our own resistances and restrictions.
- Seek out a teacher who has the ability to inspire you to practice by their demeanor and way of being in the world. Do not settle for the nearest class or teacher, as a good teacher has the power to motivate, educate, and refine.
- If you are suffering from any specific disability or ailment, consult professional advice before undertaking any of the physical practices. Meditation and relaxation should be increased in such circumstances.
- Finally, never rush practice; if time is limited, simply meditate; it is the highest form of yoga and provides the greatest rewards in the shortest amount of time.

Sun
sequences

A breath of fresh air

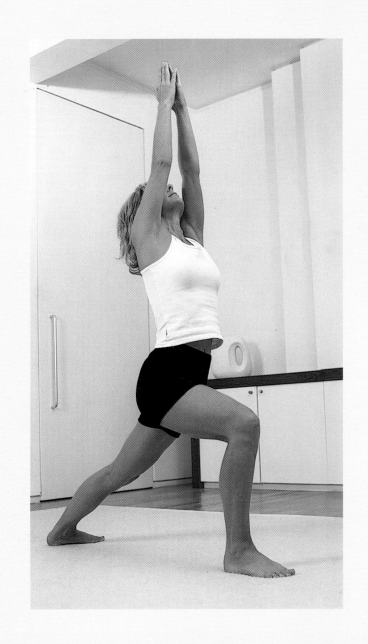

We, as inhabitants of this place we call Earth, live in a solar system. The sun is a living, breathing, pulsating entity upon which all life on Earth depends. It generates heat and light and is the source of the energy that animates us. In ancient times, the peoples of the world revered it, paid homage, and made sacrifice as a sign of their gratitude and respect. In India, the reverential practices they developed were used as a form of devotion and also as a means of channeling this life-giving energy to provide optimum health. They understood life as being a gift of the sun and, as with any gift, the greatest compliment one can pay is to use it wisely. The Sanskrit name for these exercises is Surya Namaskar, which translates as "obeisance to the sun."

Amidst the hurly-burly of the twenty-first century, we no longer seem to have the same reverential feelings for the sun. Today, we are more likely to consider the effects of the power of the sun on our skin than we are to appreciate its life-giving properties. Modern man has moved away from the innate and natural understanding of the sun as the provider of life and prime source of energy, even though science reveals that when we breathe, we are actually inhaling light, solar energy. If we can actualize this truth, we can begin to establish a deeper intimacy with the life force.

The essential ingredient necessary to reap the rewards provided by the practice of the various Sun sequences is attention, the mind being both the director and recipient of the process. The direct and controlled synchronization of the breath with the fluid, rhythmic movements of the body can only be made with sustained attention and awareness. Jerky, awkward movements reveal a lack of attention, confidence, or fatigue. Conversely, refined, attentive actions develop grace, elegance, and inner harmony. The overt and diverse movements are simply devices that challenge, educate, and enliven us. The practice of the Sun sequences is one of refinement. The benefits are an increase in flexibility, energy levels, and awareness. The Sun sequences are the foundation of all yoga practice. With regular practice they refresh our bio-energy systems and restore order, harmony, and focus to our lives.

Sun sequence I

The first of the Sun sequences originates from northern India, most predominantly from the foothills of the northern Himalayas. The movements are relatively simple and gentle, and the various actions and stretches present little difficulty and are designed to sensitively awaken and open the body. The initial action of drawing the palms of the hands together into the prayer position both indicates and establishes the quality of the form. Interestingly, it is no coincidence that every major religion uses this gesture within its various ceremonies. The simple act of pressing together the palms of the hands balances the left and right hemispheres of the brain, which establishes an attitude of equanimity and inner quiet.

The first action of exhaling and joining the palms is calm, considered, and breeds composure (see Posture 1, opposite). The following inhalation, though no less considered, is dramatic and expansive. Great care and attention are needed to ensure that the breath remains smooth and even throughout the movement. The degree and extent of the arch backward is governed by the length of the inhalation. The split second that the inhalation reaches its summit is the point where you begin moving and exhaling into the next posture. Keeping a firm grip of the lower abdominal muscles at the end of each exhalation increases the release of stale energy from the body and provides the space for a deeper inhalation. It also deepens the ability to stretch further into each posture.

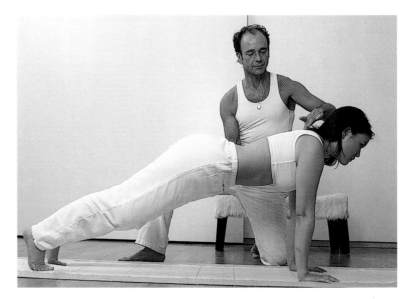

PURE AND SIMPLE

• THIS POSTURE AND THE MOVEMENT INTO IT ARE UNIQUE. IT IS THE ONLY OCCASION THAT THE BREATH IS HELD. RETAINING THE BREATH INCREASES THE INNER DYNAMIC OF THE BODY, DEEPENING THE ABSORPTION OF ENERGY INTO THE BLOODSTREAM.

• THE BODY IS BRACED FROM THE STRONG ACTION INITIATED FROM THE HANDS, UP THROUGH THE ARMS, AND INTO THE SHOULDERS. KEEP THE WHOLE OF THE BACK AND CHEST BROAD, THE ABDOMEN LOCKED, AND THE LEGS RIGID AND TIGHT. FROM THE TIPS OF THE FINGERS TO THE TIPS OF THE TOES THE BODY FEELS FIRM, STRAIGHT, AND STRONG.

• SEE ALSO POSTURE 5, OVERLEAF.

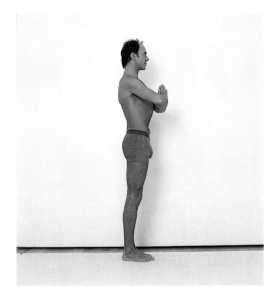
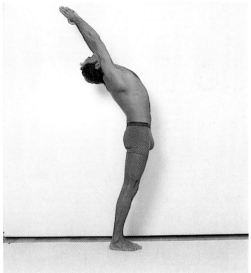
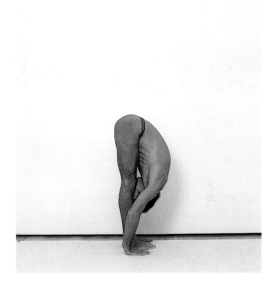

1 **Exhaling,** bring together the palms of the hands to form the prayer position. Paying attention to the smoothness and resonance of the breath, bring your awareness to the action of the intercostal muscles. Draw the lower ribs in and down, and deepen this action by tightly contracting the lower abdominal muscles. This increases the life in the legs, which should feel full and strong. Softly focus on the mid-distance.

2 **Inhaling** and keeping the palms joined, stretch the arms up and back to their fullest and begin to arch backward. Look up to the center of the forehead as the head extends back to increase the opening of the chest. Draw the spine into the body and fully expand the ribcage. Root awareness in the feet and legs to anchor the movement.

3 **Exhaling,** extend forward and down. Focus on the fingertips and follow the movement of the hands to the floor. Tightly lock the feet and legs as the fingers and then the hands touch the floor. If you cannot touch the floor and keep the legs straight, catch the calves or ankles instead. The legs must remain straight and strong throughout. At the end of this action, deeply contract the abdominal muscles.

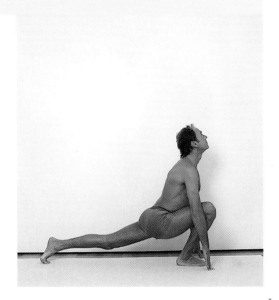

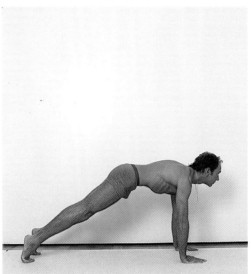

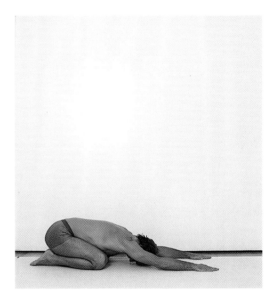

Inhaling, step back as far as you can on the left leg. At the same time, bend the right leg, drop down the hips, and lift up the trunk. Try to straighten the back leg as much as you can. Coming on to fingertips, use the arms to broaden the chest by rolling back the shoulders. Extend back the head and draw the spine in and up. Direct the gaze to the center of the forehead. (See also Pure and Simple on page 25.)

Hold the breath as you take the right leg to meet the left. Firmly push the palms of the hands into the floor, thus relieving tension in the wrists and broadening the shoulder girdle. The whole of the body is poised on the palms of the hands and the toes of both feet. Keep the legs and arms active and alive and the eyes soft, gazing into the mid-distance. The duration of this entire action should be no more than four or five seconds. (See also Pure and Simple on page 20.)

Exhaling, flip over your toes and fold backward, bringing the buttocks to the heels. Keep the palms of the hands flat on the floor and the arms straight and long. Deepen the compression of the trunk on the thighs by clenching the abdominal muscles at the end of the exhalation. Move the chin toward the chest and look down and in toward the tip of the nose.

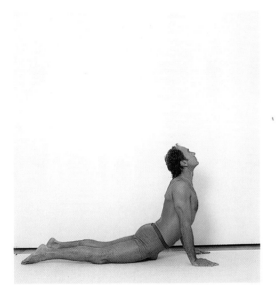
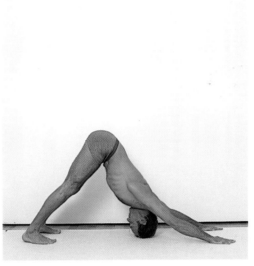
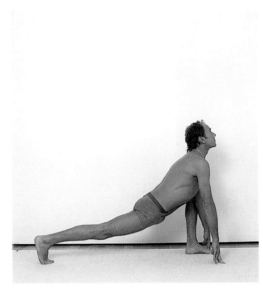

7 **Inhaling,** push forward and up, keeping the chest close to the floor. Promoting an arch of the spine from the outset of the movement, keep the elbows close to the ribs and the hands stay in the same place. As the chest approaches the hands, straighten the arms and legs simultaneously, pressing the hands, feet, and entirety of the legs into the ground. Draw the spine into the body and expand the chest fully by paying attention to the tone, quality, and resonance of the breath. Once again, look up toward the center of the brow.

8 **Exhaling,** roll over the toes and, keeping the legs and arms straight, begin to lift the hips and buttocks, carrying the chest toward the thighs. Push the heels firmly toward the floor, stretching the back of the leg muscles and contracting the front. Move the chin to the root of the neck and look toward the navel. Pay close attention to the activity of the hands. The impact of the posture originates with and from the life in the fingertips. (See also Pure and Simple on page 25.)

9 **Inhaling,** take a giant stride and carry the left foot as close to the hands as possible. At the same time, roll up on to the fingertips and lift the head and chest. Try to keep the right leg straight, lowering the left buttock as close as possible to the left heel. Look up and in.

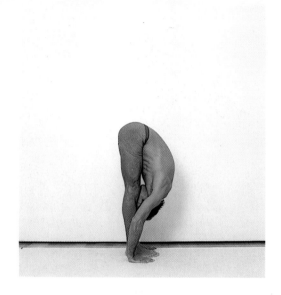

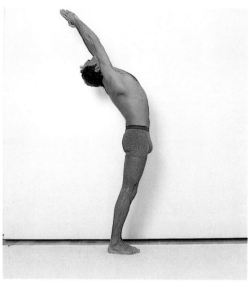

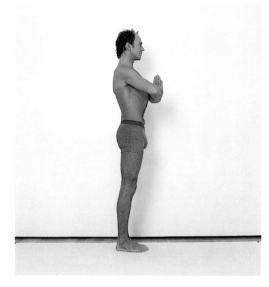

Exhaling, step forward, drawing the right foot to meet the left. From the strength and stretch of the feet, straighten the legs, keeping the hands as close as possible to their original position. Once again, if you cannot maintain contact between the hands and the floor, catch and grip the ankles or calves instead. Move the chin toward the root of the glottis and return the gaze point to the navel.

Inhaling, from the strength of the legs and feet swiftly lift the trunk and arms, bringing together the palms of the hands. Arch the back, using the arms to increase the contraction and lift of the upper spine and ribs. Extend the head backward and focus on the tips of the fingers.

Exhaling slowly and consciously, begin to return the trunk and head to an upright position. Pressing together the palms of the hands, bend the elbows and direct the heels of the palms of the hands toward the navel, contracting the lower ribs and abdominal muscles to the maximum. Rest the focal point on the mid-distance.

Repeat the sequence, exchanging left for right and vice versa.
This completes one cycle of Sun sequence I.

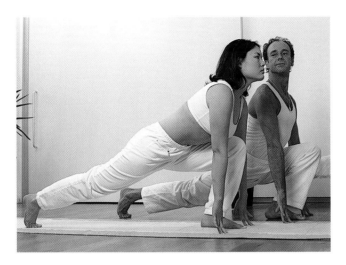

▲ PURE AND SIMPLE

• THE ACTIVITY OF INHALING AND STEPPING ONE LEG FORWARD STRETCHES ONE SIDE OF THE ABDOMINAL WALL AND CONTRACTS THE OTHER. ATTENTION SHOULD BE FIXED ON CARRYING THE LEG SOFTLY TOWARD THE HANDS; THE FOOT SHOULD REACH THE FLOOR QUIETLY, AND NOT WITH A THUD.

• THE BACK LEG REMAINS STRAIGHT AND STRONG TO PROVIDE A DEEPER STRETCH AND ALSO TO FACILITATE THE OPENING OF THE CHEST.

• SEE ALSO POSTURE 4 ON PAGE 22.

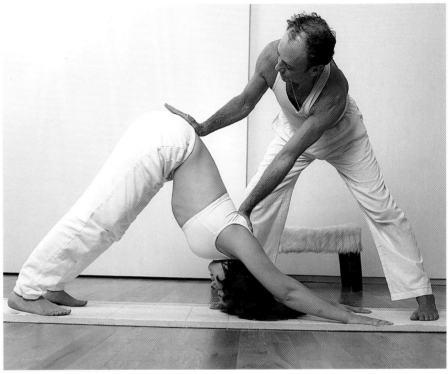

▲ PURE AND SIMPLE

• THIS POSTURE IS CALLED THE DOG POSE AND IS THE MOST IMPORTANT ONE IN THE BOOK. SPECIAL ATTENTION SHOULD BE GIVEN TO THE PLACEMENT AND ACTIVITY OF THE FEET AND HANDS. THE POWER AND LIFE OF THE POSTURE ARE INSTIGATED BY THE LIFT PROVIDED BY THE ARMS AND LEGS. THE SPINE IS THEN GIVEN TRACTION, THE SHOULDERS ARE LIBERATED, AND, BECAUSE THE DIAPHRAGM IS LIFTED INTO THE CHEST CAVITY, THE HEARTBEAT SLOWS DOWN AND THE HEART MUSCLE IS SOFTENED.

• TAKING THE CHIN TO THE CHEST PARTIALLY RESTRICTS THE AIR FLOW, WHICH QUIETS THE MIND.

• AS THE HEAD AND BRAIN ARE BENEATH THE HEART, THEY ARE IRRIGATED WITH HIGHLY OXYGENATED BLOOD. THIS IS A MOST INVIGORATING AND REJUVENATING POSTURE.

• SEE ALSO POSTURE 8 ON PAGE 23.

Sun sequence II

Evolving from the humid subtropical heat of southern India, this sequence is dynamic and powerful. The movements are more demanding and present a greater challenge than the previous sequence; however, the same principles apply. Once again, the practice is simply that of moving from posture to posture on either an inhalation or exhalation. Initially this sequence is more difficult because it involves the use of deep compression to aid in the expulsion of stale energy and the inspiration of fresh energy. This is revealed by the first jump backwards at Posture 5, where the whole body is suspended from the floor. For this action to be smooth and graceful, the muscles of the back, chest, and abdomen must tightly grip against the ribcage. The close contact of the arms with the sides of the trunk increases the pressure on the lungs, literally squeezing used energy from the alveoli and bronchioles of the lungs.

The contrasting action of springing forward into the Dog Pose at Posture 7 is done while inhaling. This requires the lower abdominal and back muscles to lock tight to carry the legs toward the hands. The strength and support provided by the hands and arms broadens the chest and shoulders, which develops the ability to draw breath into the upper lobes of the lungs. These two actions are the key elements of the sequence and may take some time to master.

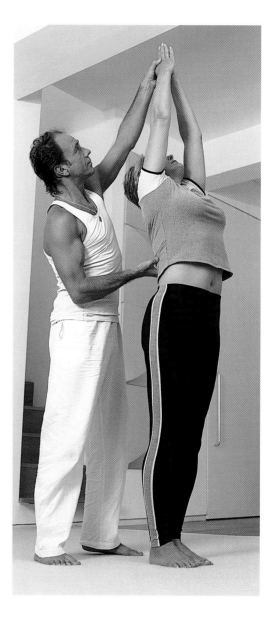

PURE AND SIMPLE

• PAY ATTENTION TO THE EQUALITY OF ACTION OF THE ARMS, THEY ARE THE INSTRUMENTS THAT MOTIVATE AND LIBERATE THE CHEST AND RIBS. IF THE ARMS ARE INACTIVE, THE CHEST AND SPINE SAG AND THE SHOULDERS ARE FORCED TO CARRY THEM.

• MAKE THE STRETCH EVEN AND COMPLETE. FROM THE ANCHOR SUPPLIED BY THE FEET AND LEGS TO THE TIPS OF THE FINGERS, THE WHOLE BODY SHOULD FEEL ACTIVE AND INVOLVED.

• SEE ALSO POSTURE 2, OPPOSITE.

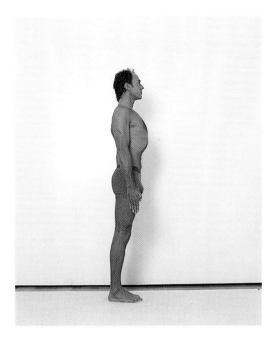 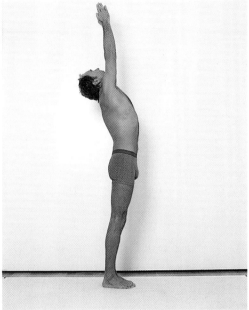 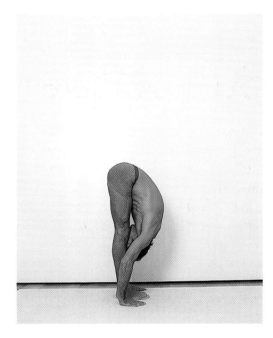

1 Exhaling, stretch the feet so that the weight of the body is distributed evenly between the ball of the big toes, the knuckle of the little toes, and the center of the heels. The feet should be together. Pull up on the knees and clench the thigh muscles against the thigh bone. Tuck the sacrum down and in, and begin to lift evenly through the spine. Broadening the back, chest, and shoulders, bring awareness into the arms, activating them right through to the fingertips. Focus softly into the mid-distance.

2 Inhaling, take the arms wide, maintaining the extension through to the wrists and fingers. As the arms reach shoulder height, rotate the palms of the hands to face the sky. Continue raising the arms to above the head. Without arching backward, draw the spine in and up. Extend the head back and, as the hands meet, focus on the tips of the fingers. Make the stretch even from the feet right through to the hands. (See also Pure and Simple, opposite.)

3 Exhaling, begin to fold forward, maintaining the strong action supplied by the feet and legs. Allow the breath to carry the trunk down toward the legs and place first the fingertips and then the palms at the sides of the feet. Tuck the chin into the chest, lengthening the back of the spine. Look softly toward the tip of the nose.

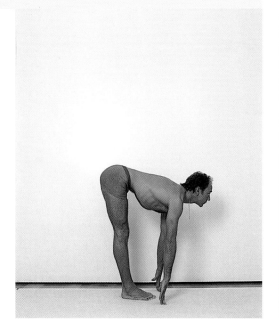
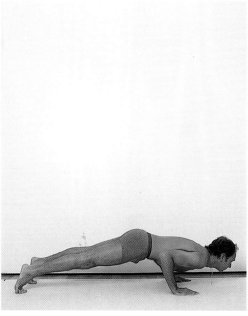
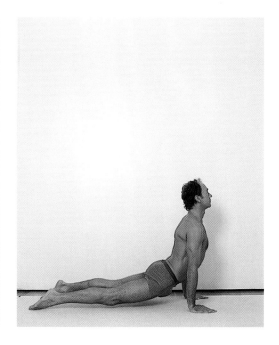

Inhaling, this movement initiates from the fingers. From palms flat on the floor, roll up on to fingertips, straighten the arms, and simultaneously raise the trunk. Arch the back as much as possible by lifting and broadening the shoulder girdle. The back does not look especially arched in this photograph, but it feels like it is. Take the head back as far as it will go and direct the eyes to the mid-distance. Both the arms and legs remain rigid throughout this movement. (See also Pure and Simple on page 31.)

Exhaling, bend the elbows and knees, take the palms of the hands to the floor, and spring back. Straightening the legs, land on the flat of the toes so that the whole body is suspended 6–9 in. (15–23 cm) from the floor. With the elbows, tightly grip the sides of the ribcage, promoting space at the back of the ribs and shoulders. Tilt back the head and gaze once again into the mid-distance. (See also Pure and Simple on page 31.)

Inhaling, push forward from the toes and roll on to the bridge of the foot. Sweeping forward and up, carry the trunk toward the hands and arch the back, opening the chest and lengthening the front of the body. The strong action of the hands and legs lifts the trunk. The thighs are off the floor with the legs straight and the rim of the pelvis close to the wrists. Grip the floor with the fingers and turn the inner elbows away from each other, broadening the chest. Draw the spine in and up and keep the neck long. Focus on the mid-distance.

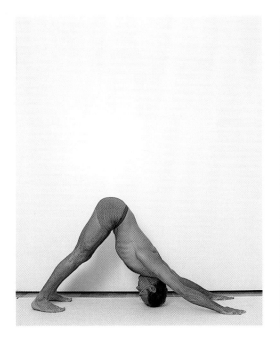

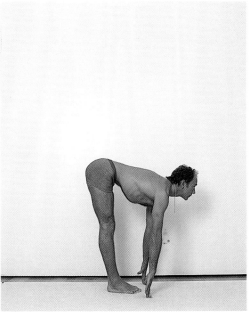

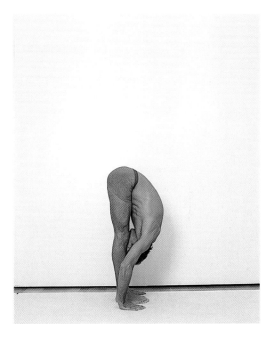

7 **Exhaling,** roll back over the toes and, keeping both the legs and arms straight, begin to elevate the buttocks and hips. Encourage the heels to meet the floor, and at the same time, carry the trunk toward the thighs. Keep the feet hip-width apart with the hands slightly wider than the shoulders. Pay attention to the pressure supplied by the fingertips, as it is from the strength of the hands and feet that upward lift is manufactured. Draw the chin to the breastbone and look toward the navel.

8 **Inhaling,** bend the knees, arch the back and spring forward, carrying the feet toward the hands. Straightening the legs, come up on to fingertips and look up toward the center of the brow, increasing the flex of the spine. Keep the arms straight throughout this movement. (See also Pure and Simple on page 31.)

9 **Exhaling,** fold forward, returning to Posture 3. Remember to maintain the strength and life of the leg muscles, as it is from this action that the spine is liberated. Move the palms of the hands to the floor and tuck in the chin. Contract the intercostal muscles and lower abdominal muscles to maximize the stretch. The focal point for the eyes is the tip of the nose.

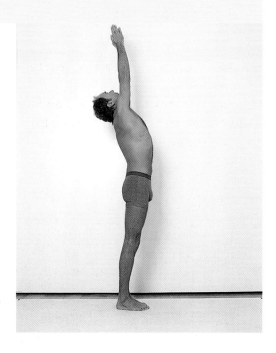

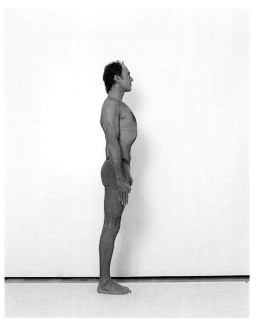

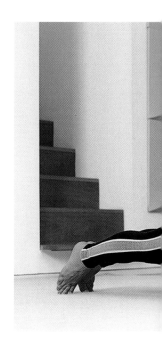

10 **Inhaling,** begin to raise the arms and swiftly lift up the head, trunk, and arms to a perpendicular position. This is a very dynamic action that starts from the strong contact made by the feet with the floor and is continued through the activity of the arms to provide the necessary force to raise the trunk and head. Slow down the arms as they reach shoulder height. Take back the head and look at the fingertips as the palms meet.

11 **Exhaling,** separate the palms and rotate them away from each other. Center the head, and as the arms reach the sides of the chest, begin to contract the rib-cage, deepening the action of the inter-costal muscles. Maintain concentration and focus upon the quality, resonance, and speed of the breath. Maximize the depth of the exhalation by firmly contracting the lower abdominal muscles and by maintaining the life and strength of the feet and legs. Focus on the mid-distance as you return to Posture 1 of the sequence.

This completes one cycle of Sun sequence II.

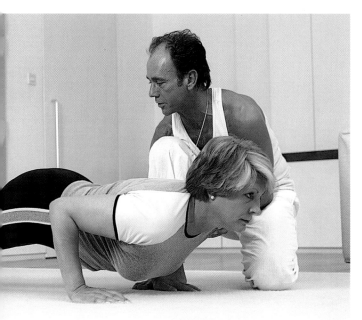

▲ PURE AND SIMPLE

• KEEPING THE ELBOWS AND UPPER ARMS CLOSE TO THE SIDES OF THE CHEST ESTABLISHES THE STABILITY OF THE POSTURE AND ALSO RELEASES THE NECK AND KEEPS THE BACK AND CHEST BROAD.

• THE LEGS MUST WORK WITH THE SAME DEGREE OF STRENGTH AS THE ARMS TO ENSURE THAT THE LOWER SPINE AND ABDOMEN REMAIN OPEN.

• SEE ALSO POSTURE 5 ON PAGE 28.

▼ PURE AND SIMPLE

• FROM THE TIPS OF THE MIDDLE THREE FINGERS, UPWARD LIFT IS PROMOTED THROUGH TO THE NECK AND SHOULDERS.

• THE FEET GRIP THE FLOOR, THE BACKS OF THE LEGS ARE STRETCHED, AND THE KNEES ARE LIFTED BY THE CONTRACTION OF THE QUADRICEPS. BOTH THE ARMS AND LEGS ARE THUS EQUALLY EMPLOYED TO PROMOTE AN ARCH OF THE SPINE AND AN OPENING OF THE CHEST.

• SEE ALSO POSTURES 4 AND 8 ON PAGES 28 AND 29.

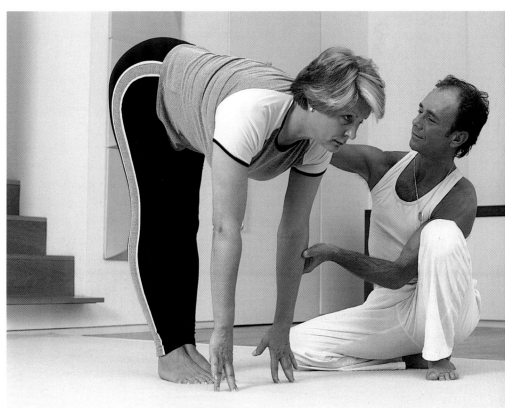

Sun sequence III

Without a doubt, this is the most challenging of the three Sun sequences. The basic form of the sequence is the same as sequence II, with the addition of two postures. The extra demands upon the respiratory system made by the inclusion of these postures teaches correct full breathing. The initial inhalation of the sequence (see Posture 1, overleaf), forces the lower abdomen to contract while the upward extension of the arms ensures that the chest lifts and the diaphragm stays open and stretched. The spine is also taught to draw in and up, furthering the education of the respiratory system.

The introduction of the second posture, where we step forward, simultaneously raising the trunk and arms, deepens the process of correction by stretching one side of the abdominal wall and contracting the other. This action not only tones the abdominal organs but breeds understanding and integration of the leg and abdominal muscles. The elevation of the arms increases lung capacity and restores elasticity to the ribs and intercostal muscles. The fingers reach up to the heavens, while the feet and legs are firmly grounded, rooted to the earth.

The objective must always be to breathe evenly and smoothly throughout each movement; from posture to posture. Labored breathing simply reveals the degree to which we have lost our ability to breathe correctly. With regular and sustained practice the difficulties presented by this sequence can be overcome and, in the process, strength, stamina, self-confidence, and a fully functioning respiratory system are developed.

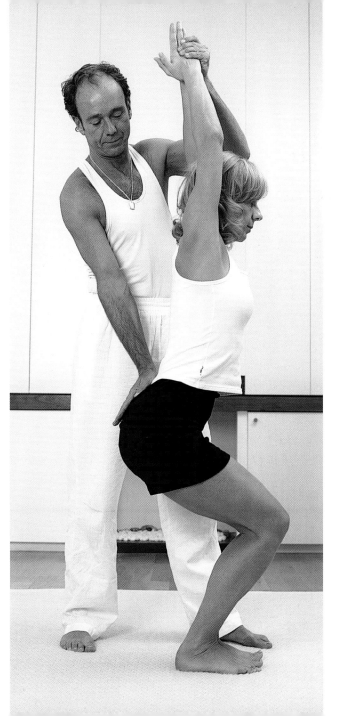

PURE AND SIMPLE

• AS THE KNEES BEND AND THE ARMS RAISE, FOCUS ON DRAWING THE TAILBONE DOWN AND IN, TIGHTLY GRIPPING TOGETHER THE INNER THIGHS. AS A DIRECT RESULT OF THIS ACTION, THE FEET INCREASE THEIR CONNECTION AND GRIP ON THE FLOOR AND THE PELVIS BROADENS, PROVIDING THE SPACE FOR THE SACRUM TO DRAW IN AND THE TRUNK TO LENGTHEN.

• ALTHOUGH THE LENGTH OF TIME SPENT IN THIS POSTURE IS ONLY ONE INHALATION, IT CAN SEEM QUITE INTENSE AND DEMANDING. PARADOXICALLY, THE INTENSITY OF THE POSTURE CAN ONLY BE MITIGATED BY BALANCING AND DEEPENING THE ACTIVITY OF EVERY MUSCLE EQUALLY AND EVENLY.

• SEE ALSO POSTURES 2 AND 14, OVERLEAF AND ON PAGE 38.

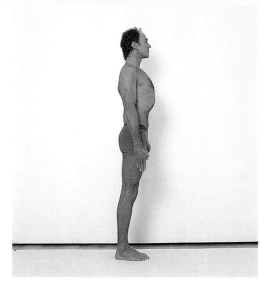

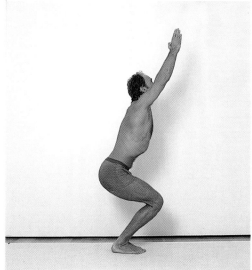

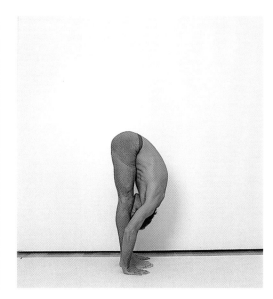

Exhaling, with feet together, arms by your sides, and standing as straight and tall as a mountain, bring attention throughout the body evenly and equally. The power of the posture comes from the strength and life of the feet and legs, which provide the motivation for the spine to lift and the chest to broaden. Keep the arms rigid and firm while the crown of the head aspires to reach the sky and the feet are firmly rooted in the ground. Gaze softly into the mid-distance.

Inhaling, bend the knees and lower the buttocks so the thighs are parallel to the ground. At the same time, bring together the palms of the hands and raise the arms forward and up. Pull the inner elbows toward each other and stretch right through the arms to the hands. Take the head back and look toward the fingertips. (See also Pure and Simple on page 33.)

Exhaling, take the chest as close as possible to the thighs and place the palms on the floor next to the feet. Begin to straighten the legs, keeping the chest close to the thighs. Move the chin to the chest and look toward the tip of the nose.

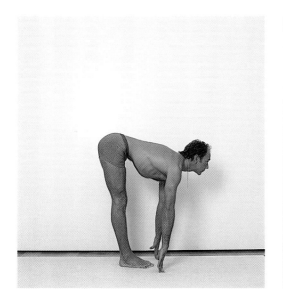

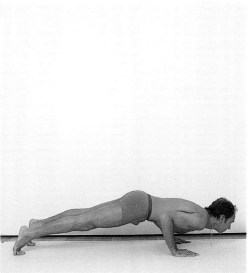

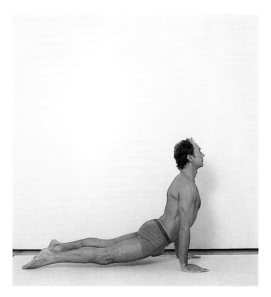

Inhaling, come on to the fingertips, straighten the arms, and arch the spine. Take the head back to increase the flexion of the upper spine and lift the tailbone high by rotating the pelvis down and drawing in the sacrum to facilitate movement of the lumbar vertebrae. Gaze softly into the mid-distance.

Exhaling, bend the knees and take the hands flat to the floor. Keeping the head up, jump back, straightening the legs so the trunk is carried toward the floor. Tightly hug the elbows against the ribs and lock the abdomen so the body is now balanced on the flat of the toes and palms of the hands. Keep focused on the mid-distance.

Inhaling, push forward from the toes on to the bridges of the feet. At the same time, push from the fingers and palms of the hands so the chest moves between the hands and the back arches. The thighs do not touch the floor at any point of this action. Rotate the inner elbows away from each other, thus broadening the chest and shoulders. Lift the head so the back and front of the neck are extended equally. Focus on the mid-distance. (See also Pure and Simple on page 39.)

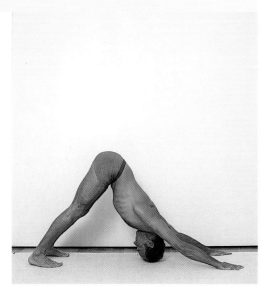

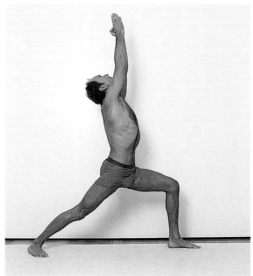

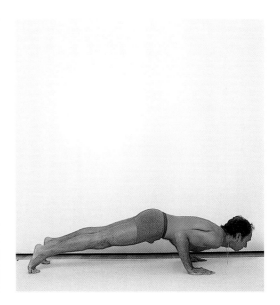

7 **Exhaling,** roll back over the toes and press the heels to the floor. The impact and lift of the trunk and hips is supplied from the pressure applied by the fingers and hands. Turn the inner wrists down and in, and broaden and open the shoulders. Lift the tailbone and move the chin to the chest to provide traction throughout the spine. Look toward the navel.

8 **Inhaling,** turn in the left foot by 60 degrees and simultaneously step the right foot between the hands. Join together the palms and raise the trunk so the thigh and trunk are at right angles to each other. The right shin and thigh also form a right angle while the back leg is straight and strong. Extend the head back as far as possible to increase the opening of the chest and the lift throughout the spine. Gaze softly at the tips of the fingers.

9 **Exhaling,** move the right leg back so the body is carried down and braced by the action of the legs and arms. Ensure that the elbows stay close to the ribs and the shoulders are broad. Also pay attention to the quality of action supplied by the hands. Focus softly into the mid-distance.

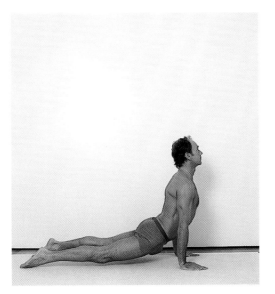

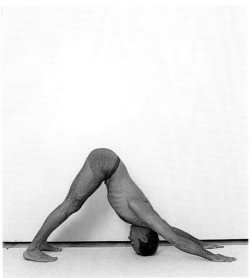

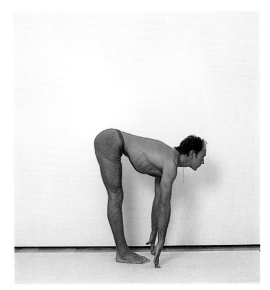

10 **Inhaling,** roll forward on to the bridges of the feet and arch the spine as the arms straighten and the trunk lifts. Both the legs and arms are straight. This activity originates in the feet and hands. The action provides the downward pressure and upward lift that facilitates an even curve of the spine and the expansion of the chest wall. Keep the chin parallel to the ground and the eyes focused into the mid-distance.

11 **Exhaling,** roll back over the toes and, stretching the backs of the legs, lift and tilt the tailbone, forward and up. Then draw the chest toward the thighs and nestle the chin at the root of the throat. Pay close attention to the equality of action between the legs and arms. The conscious application of the hands and feet provides and affords the necessary traction of the spine. At the end of each exhalation, contract the abdominal muscles as deeply as possible. Focus on the tip of the nose.

12 **Inhaling,** bend the knees, arch the spine, and look up. Keep the arms straight and maintain a close and firm contact with the ground. Spring forward, carrying the feet and legs so they arrive at the line of the hands. Straighten the legs. Coming on to fingertips, arch the spine and look up, turning the eyes to focus at the center of the brow.

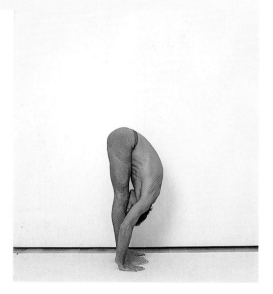

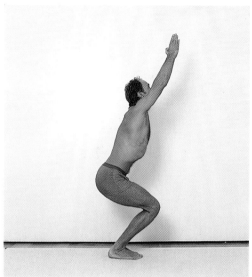

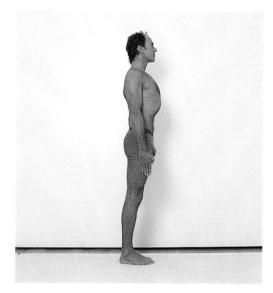

13 **Exhaling,** draw the chest down toward the thighs and press the palms of the hands into the floor. Keep the legs straight and strong, contract the front of the thigh muscles, and evenly stretch the back of the legs. Tightly contracting the lower abdominal muscles, take the chin to the chest. Focus on the tip of the nose.

14 **Inhaling,** bend the knees until the thighs are as nearly parallel with the floor as you can manage. At the same time, join the palms and raise the arms to the sides of the ears. Take back the head and focus on the fingertips. (See also Pure and Simple on page 33.)

15 **Exhaling,** begin to stand up straight, simultaneously taking the arms wide and down to the sides of the trunk. Keep the arms rigid and use to aid the contraction of the intercostal and abdominal muscles. As the hands reach the hips, draw down the buttocks and pull in the sacrum. Return the head to an upright position and gaze softly into the mid-distance.

Repeat the sequence, exchanging left for right and vice versa.
This completes one cycle of Sun sequence III.

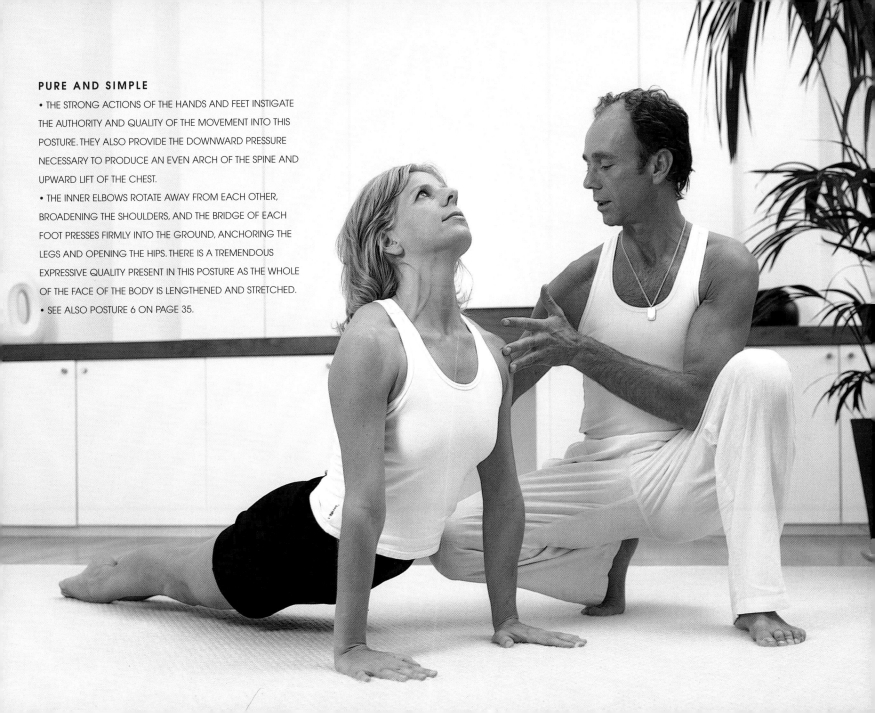

PURE AND SIMPLE

• THE STRONG ACTIONS OF THE HANDS AND FEET INSTIGATE
THE AUTHORITY AND QUALITY OF THE MOVEMENT INTO THIS
POSTURE. THEY ALSO PROVIDE THE DOWNWARD PRESSURE
NECESSARY TO PRODUCE AN EVEN ARCH OF THE SPINE AND
UPWARD LIFT OF THE CHEST.

• THE INNER ELBOWS ROTATE AWAY FROM EACH OTHER,
BROADENING THE SHOULDERS, AND THE BRIDGE OF EACH
FOOT PRESSES FIRMLY INTO THE GROUND, ANCHORING THE
LEGS AND OPENING THE HIPS. THERE IS A TREMENDOUS
EXPRESSIVE QUALITY PRESENT IN THIS POSTURE AS THE WHOLE
OF THE FACE OF THE BODY IS LENGTHENED AND STRETCHED.

• SEE ALSO POSTURE 6 ON PAGE 35.

Science reveals that when we breathe,

we are actually inhaling light, solar energy.

If we can actualize this truth, we can begin

to establish a deeper intimacy with the life

force and, consequently, the instrument

through which it shines.

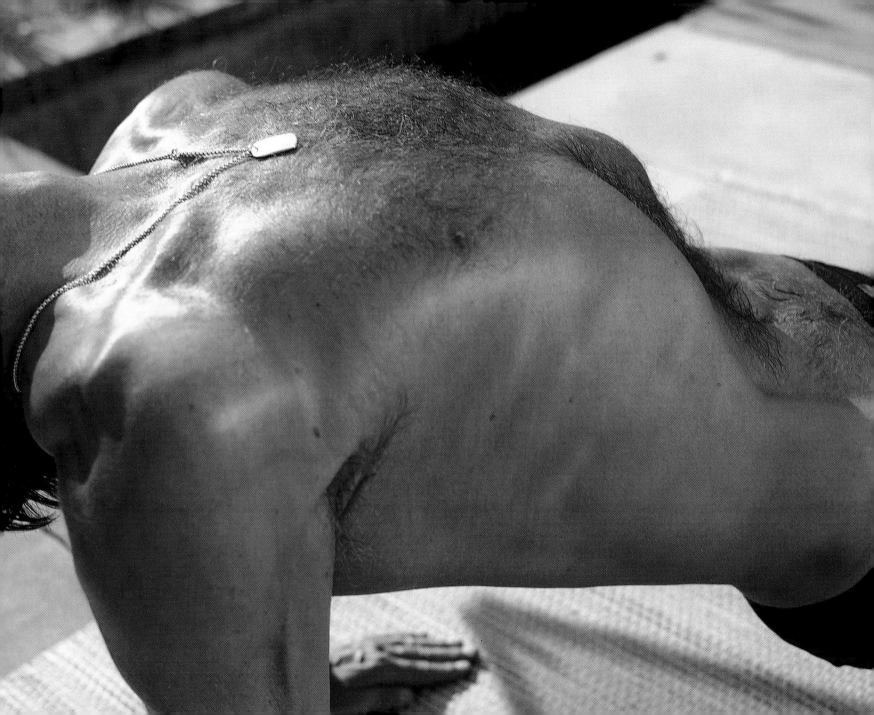

Standing sequences

A spring in your step

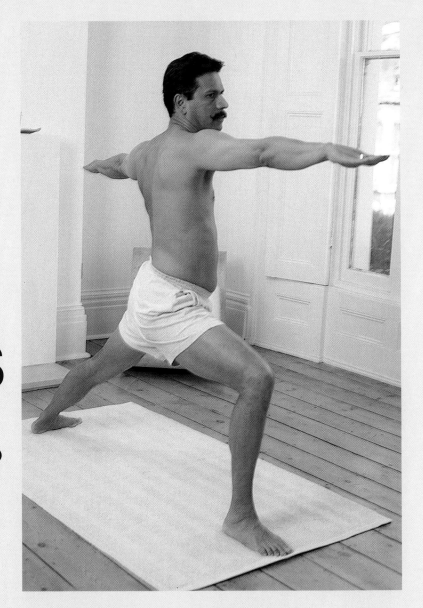

There is a common misunderstanding that yoga postures are held static and motionless. This is not the case, as if we are breathing, then we are indeed moving; movement originates with breathing and breathing is stimulated and directed by movement. As we move into the Standing postures, the principles and guidance provided by the practice of the Sun sequences still hold true, but are now applied in a different direction. The initial question raised by the Standing postures is how is that same rhythm and fluidity of the breath maintained while sustaining balance and stability? The answer is stillness, but the stillness inherent within each posture is of the mind not the body. For the mind to be drawn into the body, it needs to be still, open, and receptive. The physical demands made by the postures provide the necessary stimulus to encourage the mind to focus, and consequently to attend to the relative task.

My initial reaction to the Standing postures was overwhelming. I could not believe how difficult and intense they appeared. There seemed to be so much to think about and do, all at the same time. What seems hard to appreciate in the early stages of practice is that this is part of their strength and purpose. The conscious mind is taught to direct and enliven the various muscles and joints of the body, evenly, naturally, and dispassionately. The calm, rhythmic action of the breath carries the mind and directs energy throughout the body/posture. Gradually, the body regains accurate postural alignment and, more important, it regains consciousness—it wakes up.

As soon as we are introduced to the questions raised by the Standing postures, we realize just how difficult it is to exercise control and yet to remain focused. The mind exerts very little authority over the body; it finds it difficult to rest in the feet, legs, trunk, and arms simultaneously. The feet rebel, the leg muscles refuse to remain active and lifting, the arms tremble, and breathing becomes labored. But as a result of resolving the questions posed by the Standing postures, the director of the process, the mind, becomes vigilant, steady, and expansive. The body becomes strong, stable, and gains lightness.

Standing sequence I

The fundamental principles are all established in this, the first, standing sequence. From the firm foundation and grounding action supplied by the feet, the bones and muscles of the legs are instructed in the mechanics of support, stretch, and rotation and are thus employed to motivate and liberate the hips and spine. The movements and actions in and out of the postures are relatively simple and uncomplicated and are directed through the vehicle of the breath. Attend to using the breath to direct the movement between each posture, and also pay careful attention to the impact of the posture upon the rhythm and speed of the breath.

By attending to the depth of the contraction made by the lower abdominal muscles while exhaling, we can influence, and therefore increase, the downward pressure and life in the feet. Similarly, by focusing on the smoothness and length of an inhalation, we can further extend the spine. In this way, practice becomes progressive, breath by breath.

This sequence concentrates upon four separate and specific actions: extending the trunk laterally out of the pelvis, the arching and the lengthening of the spine, and the full rotation of the trunk and spine. By resolving these questions, minor deformities of the legs are corrected, and the feet and legs gain strength and elasticity.

This sequence of postures is best practiced as a continuance of any of the previous Sun sequences. The Dog Pose provides the perfect bridge from which to move into and through this sequence (see also page 14).

Depending on the depth and duration of your breath, hold each posture for 5 to 9 breaths, according to personal capacity and time available.

PURE AND SIMPLE

• THE TRUNK, LEGS, SHOULDERS, AND SPINE ARE ON THE SAME LATERAL PLANE IN THIS POSTURE.

• THE ANGLE OF THE FOOT TO THE SHIN AND THE SHIN TO THE THIGH ARE AT RIGHT ANGLES TO EACH OTHER, WHICH AFFORDS A STRONG STRUCTURAL SUPPORT.

• FROM THE ROTATION OF THE BACK LEG MUSCLES AWAY FROM THE FLOOR, THE PELVIS IS BROADENED AND THE SPINE MAY THEN BE EXTENDED EVENLY.

• SEE ALSO POSTURE 2, OVERLEAF.

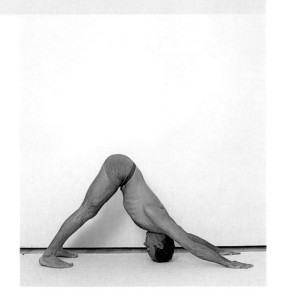

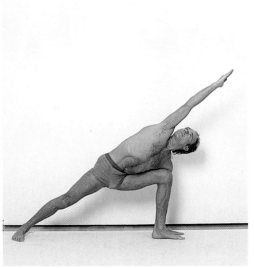

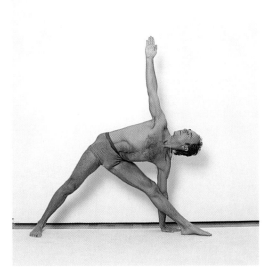

1 After completing an equal number of repetitions of any or all of the Sun sequences, **exhale** and step back into Dog Pose. Elevate the tailbone and press the heels to the ground, encouraging the trunk to move toward the thighs. Direct the life of the posture from the firm grip of the tips of the fingers against the ground. Draw the inner wrists in and down and rotate the shoulders away from each other. Align the feet so they are parallel and hip-width apart, with the backs of the knees broad and full. Contract the quadriceps and stretch the hamstrings. Place the chin firmly against the root of the glottis and focus on the navel.

2 **Inhale,** and step the left foot between the hands, opening on to a flank and, at the same time, turn in the right foot flat to the floor. Keep the left hand straight behind and in line with the angle created by the left leg. The right hand and the right foot should be on a single plane. Turn the head and neck in the direction of the extending arm, and direct the gaze to the fingertips. Breathing deeply and evenly, draw awareness to both feet simultaneously. Learn to grip the floor with the feet, as this produces stability and balance. The spine can then be motivated to move into the body and lengthen. (See also Pure and Simple on page 45.)

3 **Exhaling,** begin to straighten the left leg and, at the same time, elevate the right arm until it is vertical. Throughout this movement, fix the eyes on the fingertips. From the strong action of the feet, clench the thigh muscles against the thighs and rotate the thigh muscles of the right leg away from the ground. Tuck the root of the left leg into the hip socket by deepening the stretch of the hamstrings and the contraction of the quadriceps. Breathing freely and evenly, draw awareness into the pelvis and spine. Extend the trunk along the line of the left leg. Keep the chest broad and open, widen the shoulders, and lengthen the abdomen.

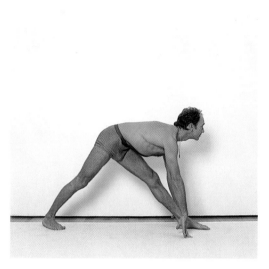
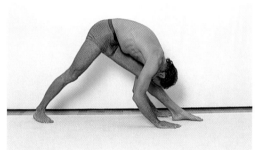
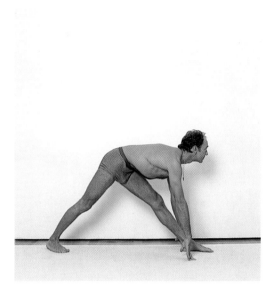

4 **Exhaling,** turn the trunk and right foot forward and lower the right hand to the floor beside the left foot and come on to the fingertips. Inhaling, lift the head back, arching the spine. Breathing freely and deeply, lift the arches of the feet by pressing the ball of the big toe and the knuckle of the little toe firmly into the ground. The front foot faces directly forward, the back foot turns in to form an angle of 70–80 degrees. This alignment allows the hips to rotate and balances the pelvis. Breath by breath, stretch the backs of both legs and lengthen the spine out of the pelvic girdle. Focus softly into the mid-distance. (See also Pure and Simple on page 49.)

5 **Exhale** and lower the trunk along the extending front leg. Bend the elbows and take the hands flat to the floor. Keep awareness and attention throughout the body, lengthening the spine with every breath. Stretch the back of the ribcage and lungs and press the chest against the front thigh. Gaze at the tip of the nose. Continue to breathe deeply, evenly, and rhythmically, contracting the root of the abdominal wall with each and every exhalation. Even though the chest is compressed, endeavor to expand the lungs to their maximum with each fresh inhalation.

6 **Inhaling,** roll back up on to the fingertips, straighten the arms, and raise the head up and back. Maintain a strong supporting action with the feet and legs, lengthening the spine and trunk out of the pelvis. Focus on the rhythm and resonance of the breath, deepening the connection and quality of action of the body. (See also Pure and Simple on page 49.)

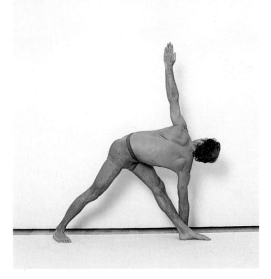

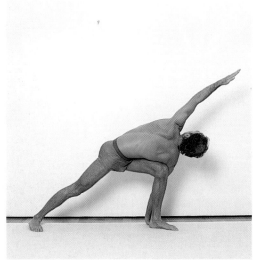

PURE AND SIMPLE ▶

• BOTH THE ARMS AND LEGS ARE USED WITH EQUAL
EFFECT TO STIMULATE AN ARCH OF THE SPINE.

• THE SHOULDERS ARE BROADENED BY THE ACTIVITY
AND UPWARD LIFT PROVIDED BY THE ARMS AND THE
FEET, AND LEGS DELIVER LIFT AND AN OPENING OF THE
SACROILIAC.

• SEE ALSO POSTURE 6 ON PAGE 47.

7 **Exhaling,** take the right hand across to the outside edge of the front foot and, if possible, place the palm flat on the floor. Inhaling, rotate the trunk, raise the other arm, and turn the focal point on to the fingertips. The legs keep the same action as in the previous posture. It is from the authority of the legs and feet that the spine and trunk are able to rotate. The arms are also fully active and alive, with the right arm lifting up out of the shoulder girdle. Breathing deeply and freely, keep the chest open, the shoulders broad, and the abdomen long. (See also Pure and Simple, opposite.)

8 **Exhaling,** bend the front leg so the thigh and shin form a right angle. Move the upper arm to point away from the body on the same plane as the back leg. Turn the head, maintaining the gaze on the fingertips. Keep the extending arm long, straight, and strong and open the shoulders and upper lobes of the lungs. Breathing can seem labored because the right side of the rib-cage is compressed and the abdominal wall rotated. So pay even greater attention to each inhalation and exhalation. Exhaling, turn and lower the upper hand to the floor and move the right hand forward next to it, stepping back into Dog Pose (Posture 1).

Repeat the sequence, exchanging left for right and vice versa.
This completes one cycle of Standing sequence I.

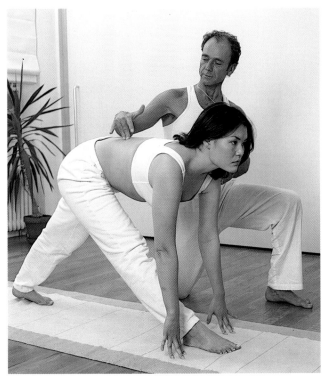

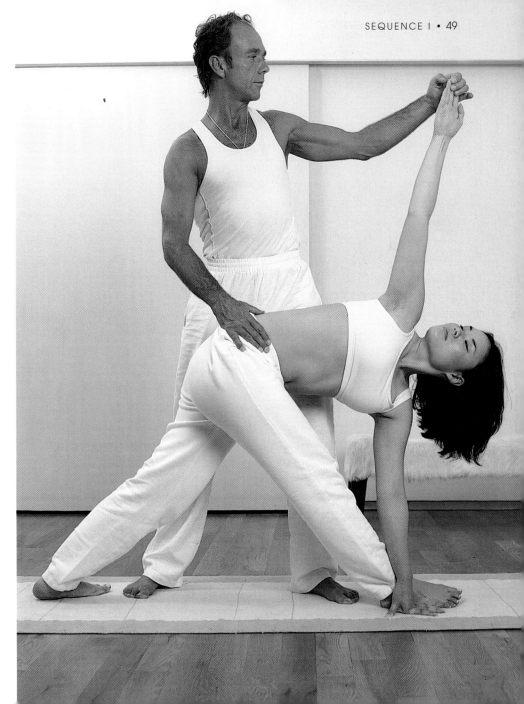

PURE AND SIMPLE ▶

• ALWAYS REMEMBER THAT THE NECK IS A PART OF THE
SPINE. THE ACCURATE ROTATION OF THE HEAD AND
NECK NOT ONLY DIRECTS THE POSTURE BUT ALSO
ENSURES FREEDOM WITHIN THE POSE.

• THE STRONG AND LIVELY ACTION OF THE ARMS OPENS
THE SHOULDERS, RELEASING THE THORACIC SPINE, AND
THE INTEGRAL ACTION OF THE FEET AND LEGS LIBERATES
THE HIPS AND LUMBAR SPINE.

• SEE ALSO POSTURE 7, OPPOSITE.

Standing sequence II

The second Standing sequence increases and deepens the activity and understanding established by the Sun sequences. The impact and importance of the breath is highlighted once more, as the essential actions of each posture can only be made by virtue of the support of the breath. This is clear from the initial movement from the Dog Pose, where the trunk is lifted and elevated by the inflation of the lungs. The influence of the movements between postures, combined with the synchronization of the breath, promotes a natural opening of the hips and spine. Freedom of the upper lung, chest, and shoulders is delivered by the strength and activity of the arms. The ratio of application between the arms and legs is identical.

In the first part of the sequence, the arms offer symmetry and balance to the trunk, encouraging deep breathing. In the final two postures, while the legs remain symmetrical, the trunk is rotated and deep breathing is challenged. The juxtaposition of the symmetrical against the asymmetrical breeds innate physical intelligence, which transforms stiff and immobile joints into light, articulate, fully functioning agents of expression. Muscle tissue softens, promoting the release of deeply held tensions and, due to an increase of blood flow throughout the body, the nervous system is stimulated and enhanced.

Like Standing sequence I, this sequence is also best undertaken as an extension of the Sun sequences and is initiated from the balancing and bridging action of the Dog Pose. The first posture of the sequence comes from the Dog Pose, and this is identical to the movement already established in the third Sun sequence, the only difference being that now the standing posture is maintained for anything from 5 to 9 breaths. Hold each of the standing postures of this sequence for the same number of breaths, without variation.

PURE AND SIMPLE

- THE STABILITY OF THE POSTURE ARISES FROM THE ACCURATE AND PRECISE ALIGNMENT OF THE FEET.
- THE LIFE OF THE POSTURE COMES FROM THE EVEN AND DELIBERATE ACTION OF THE ARMS, WHICH NOT ONLY PROVIDES SPACE FOR THE SPINE TO LENGTHEN BUT ALSO EXPANDS THE FRONT, BACK, AND SIDES OF THE RIBCAGE.
- SEE ALSO POSTURE 2, OVERLEAF.

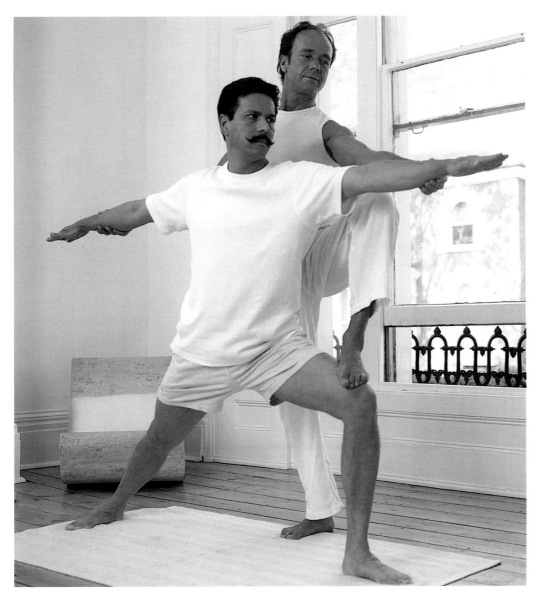

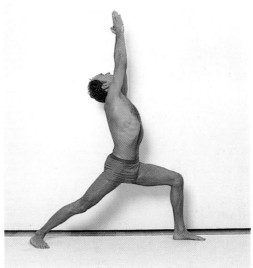

1 From Dog Pose (see Posture 1, page 46), **inhale,** turn in the right foot, and sweep the left foot between the hands. Continuing to breathe in, join the palms and raise the arms and trunk from the front thigh. Keep the back leg straight and strong. From the firm grip established by the back foot, rotate the left thigh forward, balancing the hips. Bend the front leg to 90 degrees and lift the trunk up from the root of the thigh until they are at right angles. Breathing rhythmically, bring awareness from the feet and legs, drawing in the spine and opening the chest. The abdomen is long. Extend through the arms to the fingertips. Focus on the fingertips.

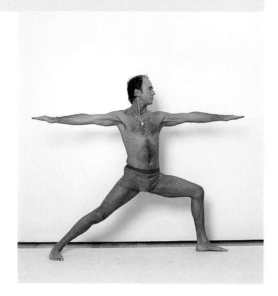

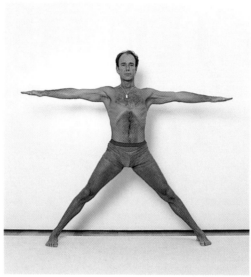

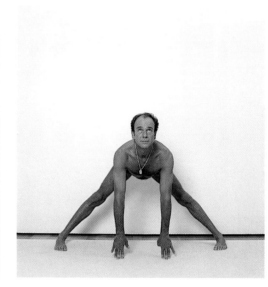

2 **Inhaling deeply and smoothly,** take the arms out wide. Turn the head and eyes to the line of the outstretched left arm. At the same time, turn the back foot out to a 60-degree angle. This action carries up to the thigh, rotating away from the floor. Continuing to breathe with full attention, draw in the sacrum and lift the spine. Use the arms to open the back of the ribcage and shoulders as well as the chest. Stretch the arms evenly, from fingertips to fingertips. Lengthen the abdomen and keep the diaphragm soft and open. Ensuring the neck is long, the head lifted, softly focus on the extending left arm. (See also Pure and Simple on page 51.)

3 **Inhaling,** begin to straighten the front leg, simultaneously turning the front foot so the feet are parallel. Keep the arms wide, active, and open. Center the head and focus on the mid-distance. To maximize the opening of the chest, back, and lungs, pay attention to evenly drawing the breath in and up, lifting the spine, and expanding the lungs and ribs. While exhaling, concentrate on contracting the intercostal muscles and lower abdominal muscles, as this not only releases stale energy from the body, but also empowers the feet and legs. Breathing is not challenged in this posture, it is promoted.

4 **Exhaling,** extend the trunk forward, taking the fingertips to the floor and arching the spine. Make this as controlled a movement as possible by focusing on the strong action of the feet and legs. Ensure that the feet remain parallel and the thigh muscles rotate away from each other. The pelvis and trunk are then free to roll over the heads of the thighs, and the sacrum moves inward. From the lift supplied by the fingers, the shoulders and back are broadened, the chest is opened, and the abdomen becomes long and hollow. Take the head back as far as possible and focus on the forehead. (See also Pure and Simple on page 55.)

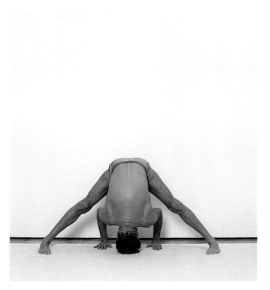

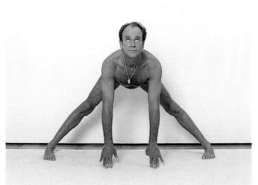

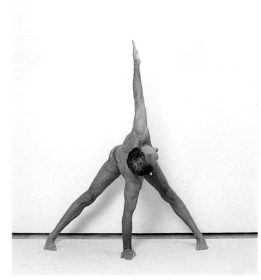

5 **Exhaling,** draw the hands back and the trunk and head down toward the floor. Aspire to rest the crown of the head on the floor, in line with the feet. Pay attention to the alignment and activity of the feet, keeping the weight evenly distributed. Translate this activity through the legs. From this powerful upward lift, the spine is lengthened and toned. Try to increase the stretch at the back of the knees and hamstrings while maintaining lift in the kneecaps and thighs. This increases the traction of the spine and lengthens the abdomen. Draw the elbows toward each other to broaden the back and shoulders. Focus on the navel.

6 **Inhaling,** sweep forward and up to the previous position. Make this movement as smooth and graceful as possible. Let the breath carry the trunk upward; maximizing the inhalation furthers the opening of the chest and increases the arch of the spine. Continue to breathe freely and deeply, noticing the flow and impact of each breath on the body. Look up and in toward the center of the brow. (See also Pure and Simple on page 55.)

7 **Exhaling,** carefully place the right hand flat on the floor directly in line with the nose. Inhaling deeply, sweep the left arm up high, simultaneously rotating the trunk, spine, neck, and head so the arms are in line. Fix the gaze on the fingertips to increase the rotation of the spine and opening of the chest. Breathing smoothly and rhythmically, extend the left arm as high as possible, creating space throughout the shoulder girdle. Weight does not settle on the right wrist, rather, the whole of the right hand is used to produce upward lift. The activity of the feet is now mirrored by the action of the hand. (See also Pure and Simple on page 54.)

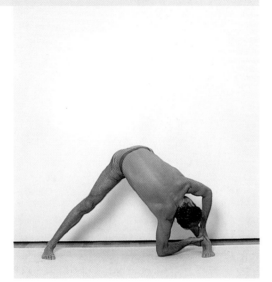

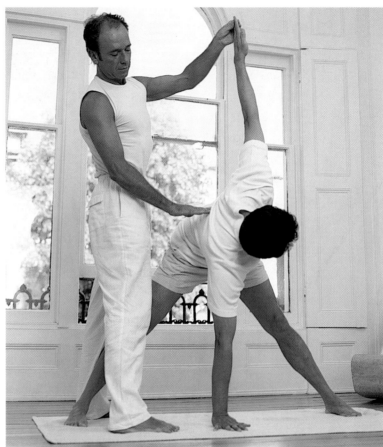

PURE AND SIMPLE

• THE HIPS AND PELVIS
ARE ANCHORED BY THE
FIRM APPLICATION OF
THE FEET AND LEGS.

• THE SHOULDERS ARE
BROADENED FROM THE
LIFT DELIVERED BY BOTH
ARMS. BETWEEN THESE
TWO COMPLEMENTARY
ACTIONS, THE SPINE IS
FREELY ROTATED.

• SEE ALSO POSTURE 7
ON THE PREVIOUS PAGE.

8 **Exhaling,** slowly lower the left arm and carry the right arm across to the left leg. Catch hold of the left shin or ankle and turn the head so the right ear is close to the left shin. Bend the arms at the elbows, broadening the back and freeing the shoulders. Keep the pelvis and hips level by maintaining the life, strength, and lift of the thigh muscles and from the grip and contact made by the feet with the ground. Breathing deeply and evenly, continue to focus on the center of the brow. Exhaling, turn on to the toes of the right foot, take the hands to the floor, and step back into Dog Pose (see Posture 1, page 46).

Repeat the sequence, exchanging left for right and vice versa.
This completes one cycle of Standing sequence II.

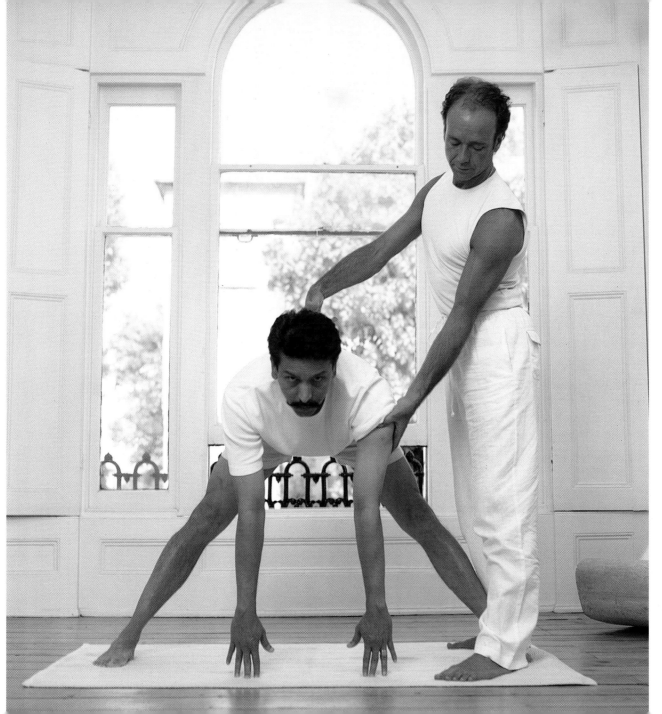

PURE AND SIMPLE

• THE STRENGTH AND
FIRM SUPPORT PROVIDED
BY THE FEET AND LEGS IS
NOW MIRRORED BY THE
EXTENSION AND ACTIVITY
OF THE ARMS.
• EQUALITY OF ACTION
THAT IS OF PARAMOUNT
IMPORTANCE TO ENSURE
THE SPINE EXTENDS
EVENLY AND NATURALLY.
• SEE ALSO POSTURES 4
AND 6 ON PAGES 52 AND
53.

Standing sequence III

The degree of difficulty and challenge is increased in this, the final Standing sequence. This is due to the extra demands made upon the legs, which are now asked to support the body individually. Because of the acute concentration needed to maintain balance, there is a tendency to hold or stifle the breath. It is therefore wise to pay careful attention to the initial postures of the sequence. Although the alternate flexing and straightening of the legs and spine can be considered to prepare the body for the later postures, the real purpose is to remind and reintroduce us to the rhythm, depth, and quality of the breath. By maintaining focus on the breath, we develop composure and a keen inner awareness. It is only this quality of mind that can instruct the body to make the slight adjustments necessary to sustain the postures. The mind becomes quick to perceive minute distinctions and acts sensitively to reestablish poise and stability. This heightens our powers of concentration and control and integrates the body/mind by exchanging the clatter of the inner dialogue for the expansive awareness of the inner eye.

Balancing postures are not only effective in revealing the disparities of the body, but also offer a most expedient remedy. Surmounting the problems and achieving mastery of the postures ensures that the correlated parts of the body work reciprocally. They develop self-confidence, independence, and equanimity.

Due to the difficulty experienced throughout the balancing postures in this sequence they are usually held for a shorter period of time: 3–5 breaths is sufficient. However, do not use this as an excuse to cut their practice short. The sequence is best practiced after completing an even number of repetitions of any or all of the Sun sequences.

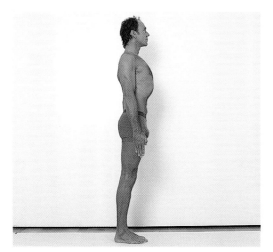 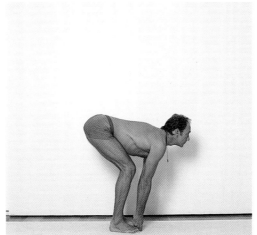 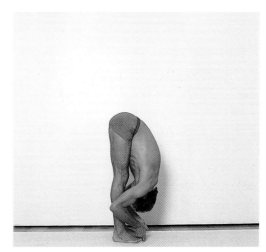

1 **Inhale** and stand straight and strong, with the feet together, gripping the floor, and the arms active and rigid at the sides. Draw the buttocks down, the sacrum in, and the chest up. Lengthen the abdominal wall and soften the diaphragm. Keep the neck long, gaze softly into the mid-distance, and aspire for the crown of the head to touch the sky. Focus on the resonance, smoothness, and impact of the breath, inhaling and exhaling freely. At the same time, work at bringing awareness into every aspect of the body, checking for areas of inactivity and over-activity. Inherent in this posture there is a dynamic, authoritative stillness. Spend enough time to access this awakened state before moving to the next posture.

2 **Exhaling,** bend the knees and crouch down, taking the chest to the thighs and the hands toward the floor. Lift up the soles of the feet and place the palms under the feet. The backs of the hands should be on the floor, with the toes close to the crease where the wrist meets the hand. Take back the head and look up, resting the focus on the mid-distance. Pressing the feet firmly on to the hands, stretch up the arms, broadening the shoulders. Breathe in deeply and increase the arch of the spine by lifting the chest and drawing in the sacrum.

3 **Exhaling,** begin to straighten the legs, drawing the chin to the chest, maintaining the connection between the chest and thighs. Bend the arms and keep the elbows close to the shins. Keep the back of the neck long and focus on the tip of the nose. Do not be overly concerned if the legs do not straighten; with application, patience, and regular practice they will. Repeat the movement from Postures 2 to 3 four or five times. Inhaling, lift the head and bend the legs, and exhaling, straighten the legs and tuck in the chin.

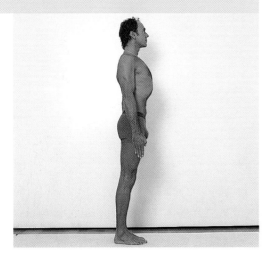 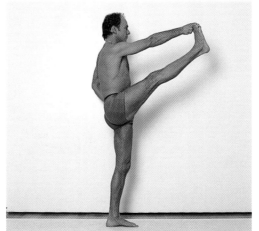 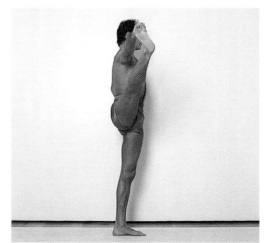

4 **Inhaling,** release the hands from the feet and stand up straight, returning to Posture 1. Establishing the inherent quality of the posture, pay attention to the increase in life and energy present in the legs, spine, chest, and arms. Utilize this fresh awareness to deepen the expansion of the whole body/mind. Focus the eyes once again softly on the mid-distance.

5 **Exhaling,** bend and raise the right leg, catching hold of the big toe with the first two fingers of the right hand. Try to keep the supporting, left leg straight and firm, with the spine drawn in and up and the chest open. Inhaling, take the left hand to the left hip and begin to straighten and extend the right leg forward and up. The fingers pull on the toe and the toe pulls firmly on the fingers, developing equality of action throughout the leg and arm. Draw back the right shoulder and, separating the shoulder blades, pull the spine deep into the body, lengthening the abdomen and the whole of the trunk, right through to the back of the neck. Breathing freely and evenly, focus on the mid-distance.

6 **Inhaling,** take the extending right leg wide and raise the left arm so that both arms are in line with the shoulders. Stay poised and balanced, noticing the rhythm and smoothness of the breath. Maintain a strong connection between the fingers and the toe, and use the right hand to increase the stretch of the leg and the foot to increase the extension of the arm. Once again, focus on the mid-distance. There is a tremendous openness and expressive quality within this posture. But watch out for how the interference of thoughts disturbs the balance.

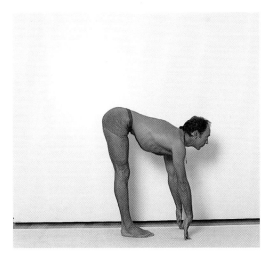 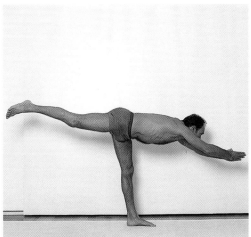 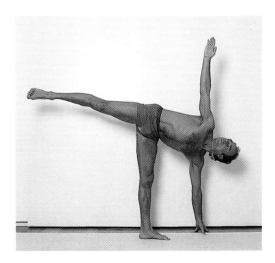

7 **Exhaling,** release the foot from the hand and, bringing both feet back together, lower the trunk, taking the fingertips to the floor. Place the hands directly beneath the shoulders, keeping the arms straight and providing an upward lift. Take the head back and focus on the center of the brow. Use both the arms and legs to deliver flexion evenly throughout the spine. The back muscles deepen this activity. Tightly grip the lower abdomen, integrating the action of the legs. Keep the body long and the diaphragm soft and open.

8 **Inhaling,** shift the weight of the body on to the left leg, and simultaneously raise both arms and the right leg so they are both on the same line as the head and trunk. The left side of the body manufactures control and support, and the right side delivers stretch and extension, heightening concentration and awareness. From the strength and support provided by the standing leg, draw in the spine and extend from the little toe of the elevated foot to the tips of the fingers of the outstretched arms. Keep attention firmly placed on the smoothness and rhythm of the breath to maintain balance. Focus the eyes softly into the mid-distance. (See also Pure and Simple on page 60.)

9 **Inhaling,** rotate the head, trunk, and back leg so they are on a flank; lower the left arm and raise the right in line with the left. Focus up to the fingertips, keeping the neck long and shoulders broad. Breathing deeply and evenly, bring awareness into both feet. Pull in the sacrum and lengthen the spine. Keep the abdomen firm and ensure the diaphragm is soft and open. Exhaling, lower the upper arm to the floor and spring back into Dog Pose. (See also Pure and Simple on page 61.)

Repeat the sequence, exchanging left for right and vice versa.
This completes one cycle of Standing sequence III.

PURE AND SIMPLE

• BALANCE IMPLIES AND
DEMANDS EQUALITY OF
ACTION, AND THIS IS
CLEARLY ILLUSTRATED BY
THE NEED FOR BOTH THE
SUPPORTING AND
EXTENDING LEGS TO
SUPPLY LIFT TO THE TRUNK.

• THE ARMS WORK
SIMILARLY TO LENGTHEN
AND OPEN THE TRUNK.
FROM THE TIPS OF THE
FINGERS TO THE TIPS OF
THE TOES, THE BODY IS
ALIVE AND ACTIVE.

• SEE ALSO POSTURE 8
ON PAGE 59.

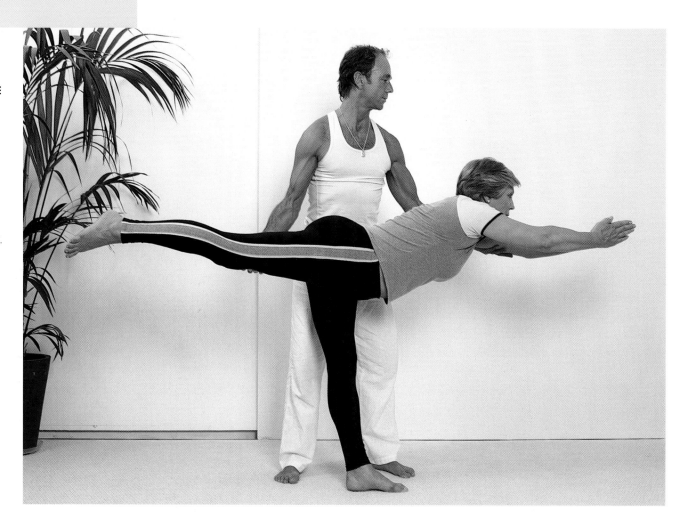

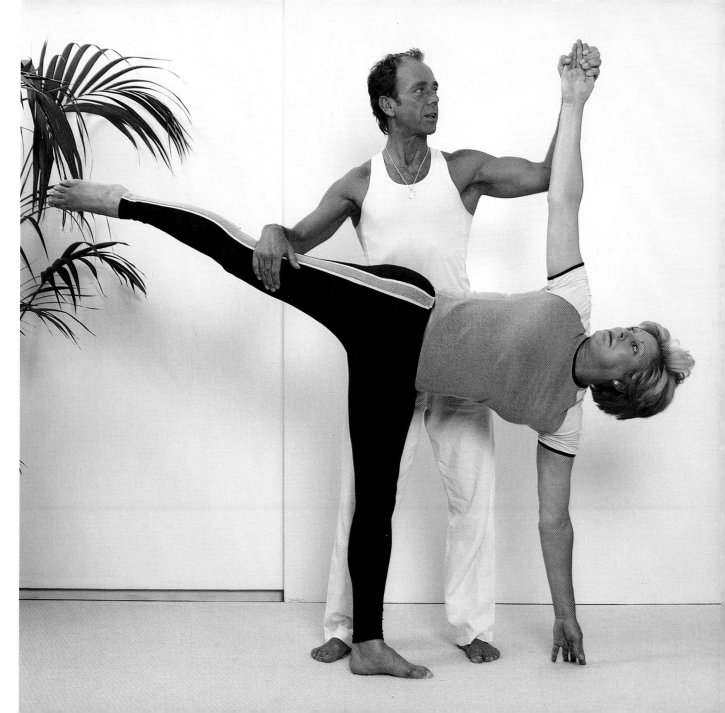

PURE AND SIMPLE

• THE ROTATION AND
OPENING OF THE PELVIS
IS REFLECTED IN THE
BROADENING OF THE
CHEST AND SHOULDERS,
THE WHOLE BODY ON THE
SAME PLANE.

• THIS IS A MOST
EXPANSIVE AND
EXPRESSIVE POSTURE,
WHICH DEMANDS
ACCURATE AND PRECISE
ALIGNMENT.

• SEE ALSO POSTURE 9
ON PAGE 59.

The juxtaposition of the symmetrical against the

asymetrical breeds innate physical intelligence,

which transforms stiff and immobile joints into light,

articulate, fully functioning agents of expression.

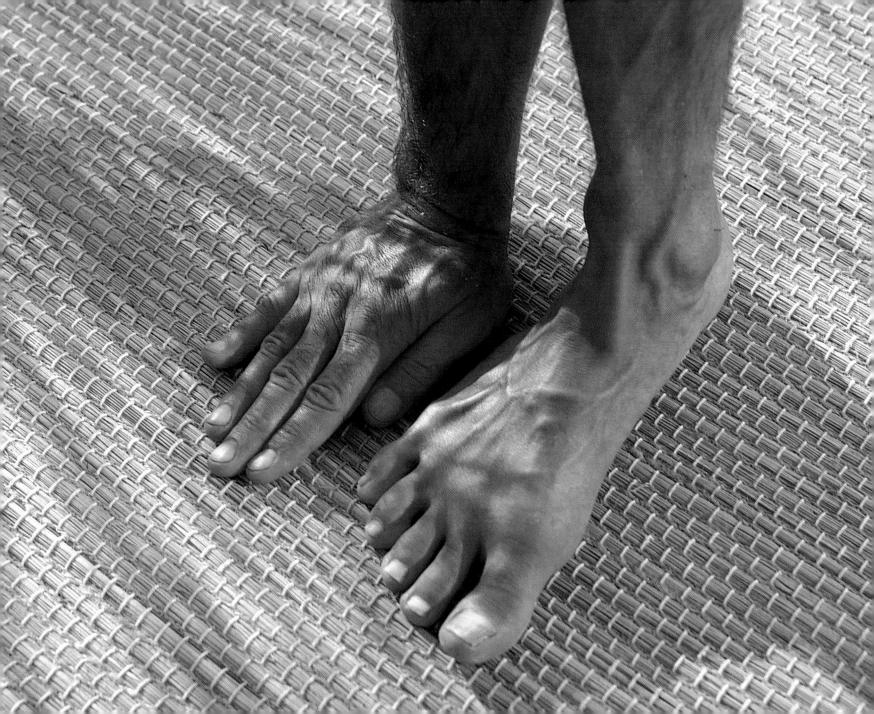

Sitting sequences

A song in your heart

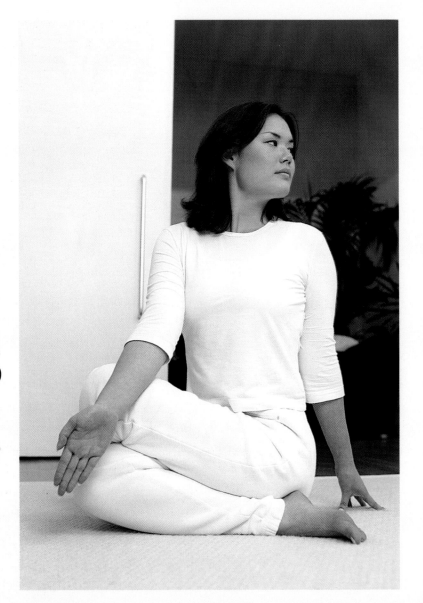

The dynamic of practice is redirected as we move to the floor for the Sitting sequences. The strength and support of the feet and legs can no longer be relied upon to generate activity and mobility of the trunk and spine. The educational process is simply furthered and refined. The sitting postures tend to be a little less intense and more subjective though no less effective. The principles established by the previous sequences hold true. It is just that now the movements in and out of the postures are mostly not as overt or obvious, although they are just as pertinent and specific. The greater range of positions and movements increases the stimulus instigated by the earlier sequences, and this breeds a deeper connection and understanding of the mechanics of the body/mind.

Although all postures exert a certain pressure and influence upon the abdominal wall, the organs of the digestive and eliminatory systems are given greater attention in these sequences. The liver, spleen, kidneys, intestines, and the other organs are alternately compressed, stretched, and rotated. Muscles, limbs, and gravity are all employed to tone organ tissue itself. Of course, the spine, lungs, and legs are not excluded from the process; rather, they are now encouraged to play a greater part in the stimulation of organ tissue.

To gain the maximum benefits offered by regular practice, always direct attention to manufacturing a strong grip with the lower abdominal muscles at the end of each exhalation, and releasing the diaphragm to enable the lungs to fully expand with each fresh inhalation. This not only animates the postures, but also promotes space within the relative confines of each posture. Natural deep breathing is the experience of expansion and contraction, and this experience is used here to influence the rest of the body. If one aspect of the body is in a state of contraction, another must be expanded. This is the basic principle of peristalsis. An increase in the peristalsis of muscle and organ tissue results in the release of tension and fatigue and the restoration of inner order and good health.

Sitting sequence I

There are three aspects of this sequence that are immediately evident. The first is the initial jump from the Dog Pose, which breeds strong arms, shoulders, and abdominal muscles. This exhilarating action trains the lower back muscles and abdominal muscles to work equally and in conjunction with each other. The second is the attention given to the two main girdles of the body: the shoulders and pelvis. Through the device of the interlocked legs, the pelvic girdle is broadened, opening the lower back and refreshing the hips. In contrast, through the diversity of the actions of the arms and spine, the shoulders and chest are developed, and tension and discomfort are relieved.

As with most of the sequences, the right side of the body is attended to first and then the left. Because of the degree of influence this places upon each particular side of the body, a powerful balancing action is needed. This is the third distinct element of the sequence. The jump back into the Dog Pose at the end (see Posture 8) has the effect of snapping the body back into alignment. This not only ensures safe practice, but is an important element in the furtherance of the education of the muscles of the body into the nature of support. The body is used as its own gymnasium; no external weights or instruments are necessary.

The individual postures of this sequence should be held for between 4 and 6 breaths, depending on personal capacity and level of experience.

PURE AND SIMPLE

• INCREASING THE PRESSURE BETWEEN AND ELEVATION OF THE ENTWINED ARMS BROADENS THE SHOULDERS AND LENGTHENS THE WHOLE OF THE TRUNK. THIS ACTION IS REFLECTED IN THE LOOSENING OF THE HIPS AND THE LIFT AND LIFE IN THE SPINE.

• SEE ALSO POSTURE 3, OVERLEAF.

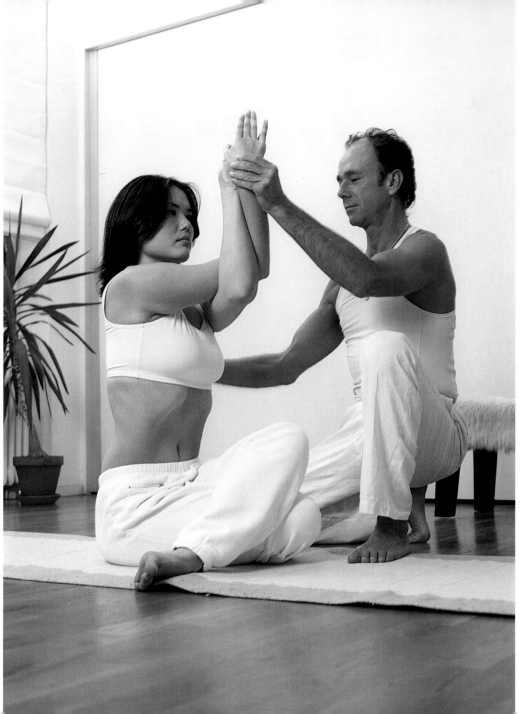

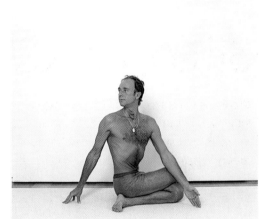

Inhaling, from Dog Pose (see Position 1, page 46), spring forward to a sitting position taking the right leg over the left so the knees meet and the feet are on either side of the hips. Exhaling deeply, rotate the trunk, neck, and head to the right. Turn the eyes in the direction of the twist and look into the corners of the eye-socket. Sweep back the right arm and press the fingers into the floor to provide upward lift. Move the left arm across the right thigh and use it as a lever to deepen the twist and to increase the rotation and opening of the shoulders and chest. Breathing deeply and rhythmically, keep the upward lift of the spine. Ensure that the diaphragm stays soft and open. Exhaling, return the trunk and arms to the center.

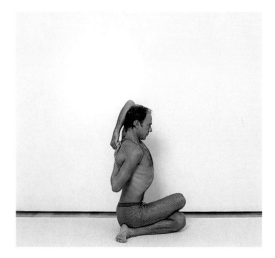

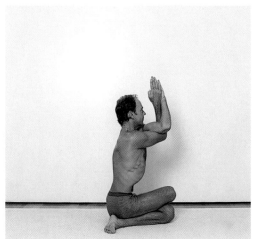

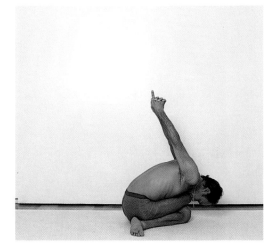

Inhaling, raise the right arm straight and high. From here, sweep it wide, round, and back so the back of the hand rests high up the spine, close to the root of the neck. On the same breath, raise the left arm back and over the left shoulder, and clasp the hands. The upper hand pulls the lower and the lower hand pulls the upper. Paying attention to the resonance and quality of the breath, use the hand grip to increase the elevation of the thoracic spine, broadening the chest and expanding the ribcage in the process. Brace the neck and back of the head against the upper arm and focus on the tip of the nose. Exhaling, release the arm lock.

Inhaling, extend the right arm forward, straight and in line with the shoulder. Breathing out deeply, take the left arm across and over the right arm so the left elbow rests on top of the right. Now bend the right arm and clasp the right hand with the left. Place the palms together and, breathing evenly and deeply, lift the elbows to chin level, simultaneously lifting the spine. Tightly squeeze together the elbows translating this action into the shoulder girdle, which also broadens and opens. Remain focused on the tip of the nose. Exhaling, release the arm lock. (See also Pure and Simple on page 67.)

Inhaling, sweep both arms back behind the body and tightly clasp together the hands. Straightening the arms, open the chest and draw the spine in and up. Exhaling, extend forward over the upper thigh, taking the chin close to the chest. Raise the arms straight and as high as possible. Continue to breathe evenly and deeply, deepening the strong action of the arms and hands, breath by breath. The eyes stay resting on the tip of the nose. Inhaling, release the arm lock and sit up. (See also Pure and Simple on page 70.)

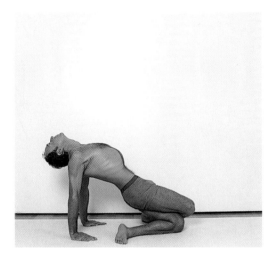

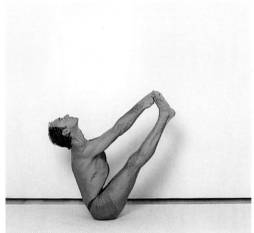

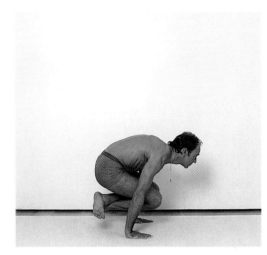

Exhaling, sit up straight and tall and extend the arms back so the fingertips touch the floor. Inhaling, roll back on to the palms of the hands and, at the same time, raise the buttocks and trunk and extend the head back as far as it will go. The focal point of the eyes now moves to the center of the brow. Tightly pull together the knees to increase the opening of the hips and also to enable the sacrum and lumbar vertebrae to draw into the body. From the strength and lift provided by the hands and arms, fully expand the chest, broaden the shoulders, and stretch the diaphragm. Exhaling, release from this posture, returning to an upright position.

Inhaling, undo the legs and take the knees to the chest with the feet together and off the floor. Take the arms to the sides of the bent legs and, with the first two fingers of each hand, catch hold of the neck of the big toes. Exhaling, straighten the legs and arms, making sure the toes pull on the fingers with as much authority as the fingers pull on the toes. Inhaling, take the head back and focus on the center of the brow. Continue to breathe rhythmically, maintaining balance by locking the lower abdomen and drawing the spine into the body. The action of the legs and arms are equal and opposite. Pull back the hands and arms and extend the legs forward and up. Exhaling, release the feet. (See also Pure and Simple on page 71.)

Exhaling, cross the legs so the left shin sits on top of the right calf and put the palms of the hands flat on the floor. From the strength of the fingers and hands, straighten the arms and roll forward, lifting the feet, legs, and buttocks off the floor. This requires determined, concentrated effort and promotes a firm contraction of the inter-costal muscles and ribs. The lower abdominal muscles contract, and the legs are literally supported and carried by the root of the abdominal wall.

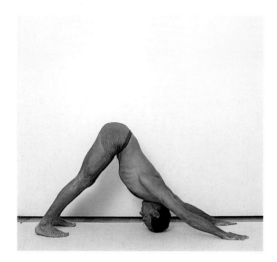

On the same breath, sweep the whole of the body back through the hands. Move the chin to the chest and look down to the tip of the nose; the breath carries the trunk and legs back into Dog Pose. This is quite a tricky movement and requires determination, focus, and application. Do not despair, though; everyone struggles with this action initially.

**Repeat the sequence, exchanging left for right and vice versa.
This completes one cycle of Sitting sequence I.**

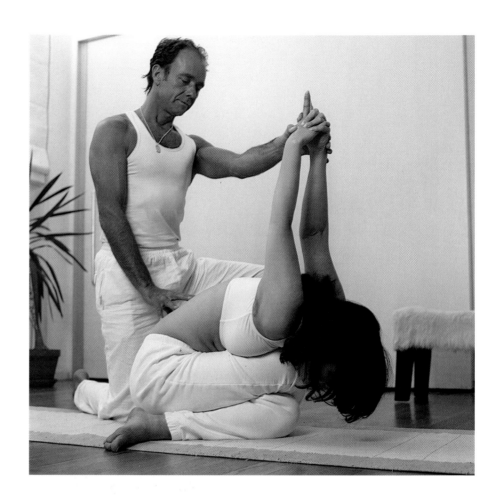

PURE AND SIMPLE

• IT IS FROM THE FIRM GRIP OF THE FINGERS AND THE CLOSE PROXIMITY OF THE PALMS THAT THE ARM MUSCLES ARE EQUALLY STRETCHED AND TONED.

• THE FORWARD EXTENSION OF THE SPINE STIMULATES THE NERVES OF THE BACK AND INCREASES BLOOD CIRCULATION IN THE PELVIS AND HIPS.

• SEE ALSO POSTURE 4 ON PAGE 68.

PURE AND SIMPLE

• AFTER THE MANIPULATION OF THE ARMS AND THE CONSTRICTION AND MAINTENANCE OF THE LOCK OF THE LEGS, THIS POSTURE PROVIDES A MARVELOUS REFRESHMENT FOR THE ARMS AND LEGS.

• THE INNER SPINAL AND ABDOMINAL MUSCLES WORK IN UNISON, AND THE WHOLE BODY IS POISED ON THE SITTING BONES.

• SEE ALSO POSTURE 6 ON PAGE 69.

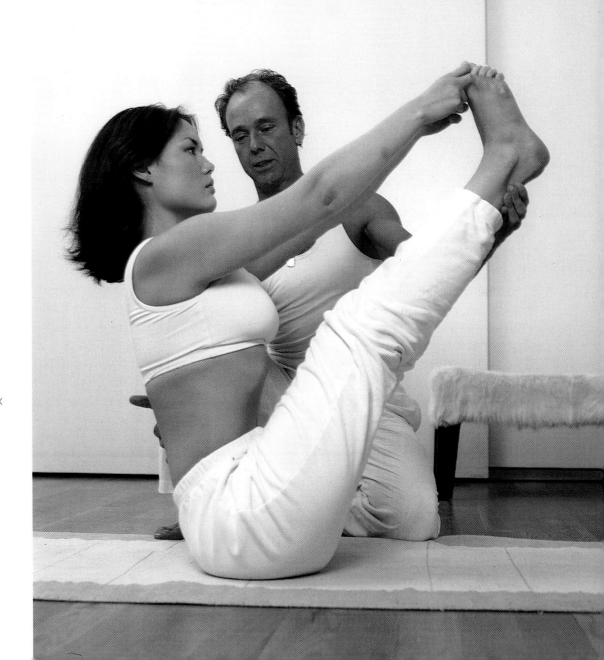

Sitting sequence II

This series of postures concentrates on generating the necessary stimulus to the spine to exchange our deeply held latent tensions for fresh vibrant energy. We carry a tremendous amount of locked energy in the lower back, hips, and shoulders, which impedes and restricts our mobility and the flow of energy through the body. This has an obvious and debilitating effect upon our everyday lives. The release of this energy opens up a deep reservoir of inherent, internal vigor.

The fulcrum of the sequence is the Locust position (see Posture 4), which is so called because, just as a locust has an appetite that cannot be satisfied, the practice of these various back arches gives us an insatiable appetite for life.

The essential action of all back bends is the expansion of the chest wall and the contraction of the spine. Care and attention must be made to produce deep, rhythmic breathing, as even though the chest and lungs are expanded, breathing can become labored and forced. This is because the generative action of the posture comes from the lower abdomen, which is trained to lift and support weight in a state of stretch. This develops deep tensile strength of the abdominal muscles and stimulates the digestive tract and stokes the gastric fire. The impact of the alternate raising of the legs, chest, and even the whole body is rooted from the pubis, which is approximately 2–3 in. (5–7.5 cm) beneath the navel. It is from this point that the chest, legs, and spine are activated. The final two postures on page 76 ask further questions about the abdominal muscles, which has the effect of both deepening their integrity and tone and of establishing balance to the body/mind.

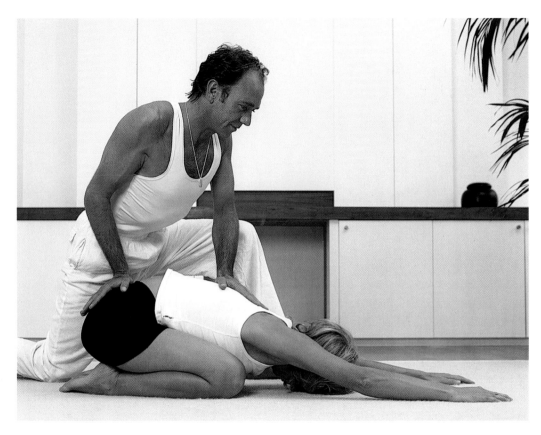

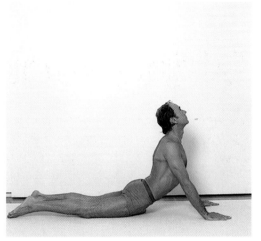

PURE AND SIMPLE

• ALTHOUGH THIS POSTURE MAY SEEM TOO SIMPLE TO HAVE ANY BENEFIT OR EFFECT, IT SHOULD NOT BE DISREGARDED. THE COMPRESSION OF THE FACE OF THE BODY AND THE LENGTHENING OF THE SPINE SOOTHES THE NERVES OF THE TRUNK AND AIDS IN THE ABSORPTION OF FRESH, VITAL ENERGY AND THE EXPULSION OF STALE, USED ENERGY.

• THIS IS AN INTROSPECTIVE AND REFRESHING POSTURE, WHICH IS MOST WELCOME AFTER THE INTENSITY OF THE EXPRESSIVE BACK ARCH.

• SEE ALSO POSTURE 2, OVERLEAF.

Inhaling, place the palms under the shoulders so the fingers are in front of the shoulders and the roots of the wrists meet the shoulders. Pressing the fingers firmly into the ground, begin to straighten the arms. Keep the elbows close to the ribs and the pelvis against the floor, and arch up and back. The strength and life of the arch depends upon the pressure produced by the feet and legs, and the hands and arms. Rotate the inner elbows away from each other to increase the opening of the chest and encourage the spine to lift higher into the body. Tilt back the head and look to the center of the brow. Exhaling, lie down flat.

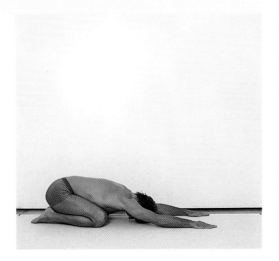

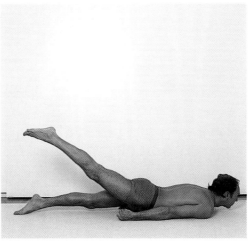

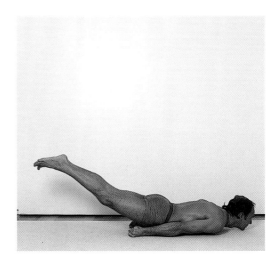

Exhaling, bend the knees and roll backward, carrying the buttocks to the heels. The knees broaden a little so the sides of the ribs nestle on to the inner edges of the thighs. Keep the arms straight and alive throughout the sweep back so the arms broaden and anchor the shoulders, just as the buttocks and legs lengthen the lower back and open the hips. Paying attention to the change in the speed and depth of the breath, also notice the strength of the expansion and contractions of the heart wall. Remain in the posture until the pulse has returned to normal and turn the eyes to gaze softly down to the tip of the nose. Inhaling, return to lying face down on the floor. (See also Pure and Simple on page 73.)

Exhaling, stretch the body out straight and long, forming the hands into fists at the sides of the hips. Press the fists, thumb side down, into the floor. Raise the right leg, extending it evenly right through to the little toe. Firmly push the downward leg, the hands, and lower abdominal muscles into the floor. Fix the pelvis to the ground, lengthen the face of the body, widen the shoulders, and focus softly into the mid-distance. Exhaling, lower the lifting leg.

Inhaling deeply, raise the feet and legs off the ground as high as possible. Press together the inner edges of the legs and stretch evenly through to the feet and toes. From the strong action supplied by the hands and lower abdominal muscles, draw the spine into the body and lengthen the face of the body, keeping the diaphragm soft and open. Breathing as deeply as possible, extend through to the front of the neck, resting the chin on the floor. Gaze softly into the mid-distance. Exhaling, return the legs to the floor.

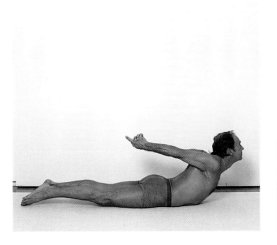

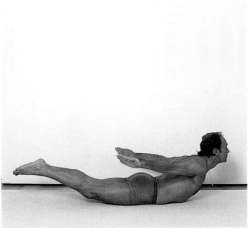

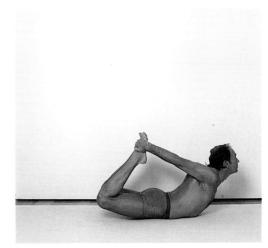

Inhaling, raise the head, trunk, and arms and tightly clasp the hands at the back of the body. Straighten the arms, pulling the inner elbows toward each other and carry the head back. Exhaling, compress the front of the legs and the bridge of the foot firmly into the floor. Contract the lower abdomen and draw the sacrum into the body. Expand the front of the body, contract the back. Breathing deeply and rhythmically, focus the eyes at the center of the brow. Exhaling, lower the trunk back to the floor.

Inhaling, sweep the arms, legs, trunk, and head up and back. Keep the arms wide and active with palms outstretched. This activity expands the lungs, chest, and shoulders and invigorates the spine. Pull together the legs so they feel full and strong, pull in the sacrum, and lengthen the front of the body. Carry the stretch of the front of the body up through the front of the neck. Direct the focal point toward the center of the brow. Exhaling, lie down flat.

Inhaling, bend the legs and, taking the hands back, catch the feet or shins and lift up, arching the spine and expanding the chest. Take back the head, increasing the opening of the upper spine, and keep the eyes focused on the center of the forehead. Pay attention to the equality of action of the body and the rhythm, resonance, and depth of the breath, increasing the lift of the legs and the chest with every breath. Exhaling, release the hands and feet and lie down and roll on to the left-hand side of the body. (See also Pure and Simple on page 77.)

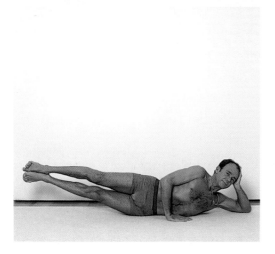

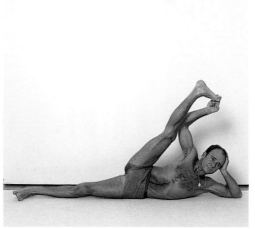

Inhaling deeply, extend the left arm straight out along the floor, in line with the rest of the body. Bend the left arm and take the palm to the temple, with the middle finger pressing on to the fontanelle (the crown of the head). Place the right hand palm down, close to the solar plexus. On an exhalation, raise both legs from the floor, tightly gripping together the inner edges of the legs. Lengthen the left-hand side of the trunk and, breathing deeply and evenly, gaze softly into the mid-distance. Exhaling, lower the legs back to the floor.

Inhaling, bend the upper leg and catch hold of the neck of the big toe with the first two fingers of the free hand. Exhaling, begin to straighten the upper leg, ensuring that the toe pulls on the fingers with as much authority as the fingers pull on the toe. The outside edge of the downward leg presses firmly into the ground, activating and integrating the action of the inner thigh and abdominal muscles. Opening the back of the knee of the extending lifting leg, draw the foot down toward the head. The gaze point for the eyes is mid-distance. On an exhalation, take the body flat to the floor and lift back into Dog Pose. (See also Pure and Simple, opposite.)

**Repeat the sequence, exchanging left for right and vice versa.
This completes one cycle of Sitting sequence II.**

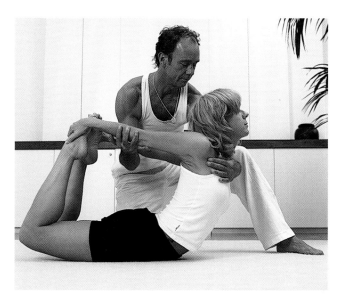

PURE AND SIMPLE

• PRESSING THE OUTSIDE EDGE OF THE DOWNWARD LEG INTO AND AGAINST THE FLOOR ANCHORS THE POSTURE AND INTEGRATES THE ACTION OF THE INNER THIGH MUSCLES WITH THE ABDOMINAL MUSCLES. THIS ACTION IS CONTRASTED BY THE LIFT AND EXTENSION OF THE UPPER LEG.

• CONCENTRATION UPON THE SUBTLE INNER ACTIONS IS HEIGHTENED BY THIS POSTURE.

• SEE ALSO POSTURE 9, OPPOSITE.

PURE AND SIMPLE

• BOTH THE ARMS AND LEGS ARE EQUALLY EMPLOYED TO PROMOTE AN EVEN ARCH OF THE SPINE.

• FROM THE ROOT OF THE ABDOMEN, THE ENTIRE FRONT AREA OF THE TRUNK IS EXPANDED TO THE MAXIMUM. THIS FULL AND PROUD EXPANSION TONES THE NERVES OF THE FRONT OF THE BODY.

• SEE ALSO POSTURE 7 ON PAGE 75.

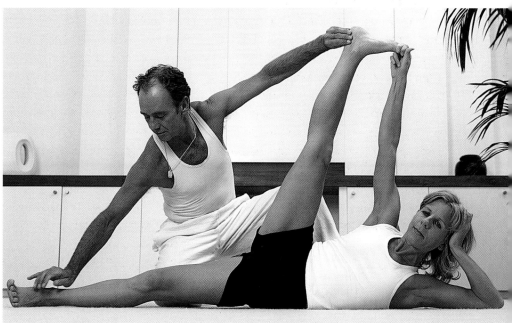

Sitting sequence III

Balance, expansion, contraction, rotation, and stretch are all given equal attention in this series of movements and postures. All of the vital organs of the body, including the heart, are massaged and stimulated. The spine gains elasticity and is rejuvenated by the forward, lateral, and backward movements supplied through the various postures. Deep rhythmic breathing is alternately encouraged and challenged in order to develop and reawaken the natural intelligence of the lungs, ribcage, and spine.

The compression of the front of the body in forward bending offers resistance to the muscles of the chest and abdomen, which consequently strengthens them and increases the inner dynamic of the lungs. The back of the lung is simultaneously expanded, developing flexibility of the back of the ribs and spine. In the counter-pose, the whole of the face of the body is lengthened and stretched, and the muscles of the back, arms, and legs tighten to provide support and upward lift.

In the early stages of practice, it can seem that the accent of these postures is mainly directed to the acute stretch of legs. However, we must realize from the outset that the legs and arms are simply the instruments used to enliven and stimulate the entire body/mind.

The final posture of the sequence (on page 82) is as formidable as it is rewarding. Allied to the lateral twist of the spine, it develops and strengthens the lower back and breeds a deep connection and important association with the abdominal muscles. Far superior to sit-ups, the regular practice of these postures promotes strength, flexibility, and a firm, resolute will.

PURE AND SIMPLE

• THE ACTIONS OF THE LEGS AND ARMS ARE OF EQUAL IMPORTANCE, AND BOTH ARE EMPLOYED TO RESTORE NATURAL FLEXIBILITY TO THE SPINE.

• THE EXTENSION OF THE TRUNK DOWN THE FRONT OF THE THIGHS MASSAGES AND STRENGTHENS THE HEART MUSCLE AND DEEPENS THE OPENING OF THE PELVIS, THEREBY INCREASING THE FLOW OF HIGHLY OXYGENATED BLOOD TO THE REPRODUCTIVE ORGANS.

• SEE ALSO POSTURE 2, OVERLEAF.

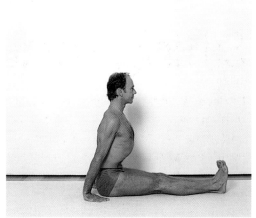

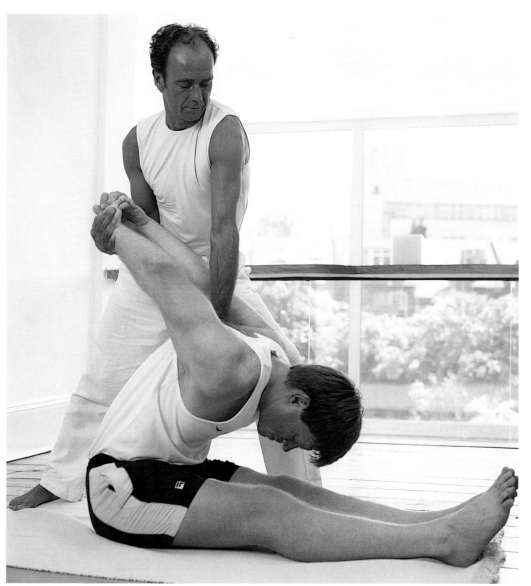

From Dog Pose, **inhaling**, spring forward, carrying the legs and buttocks to the floor coming into a sitting position. Inhaling, straighten the legs flat on the floor and together. Press the palms flat into the floor on either side of the hips and draw the spine in and up. The whole of the back of the legs push firmly into the ground and the feet are active and alive, the toes of both feet fanned open. Breathing deeply and purposefully, rotate the inner elbows away from each other, opening and broadening the shoulders and chest. Lengthen the abdomen, spine, and neck, and gaze into the mid-distance.

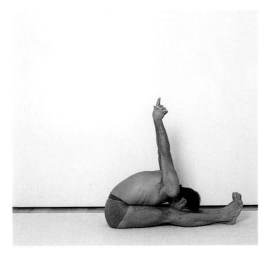 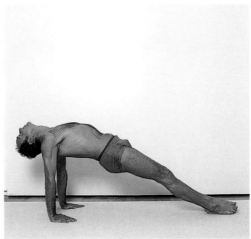 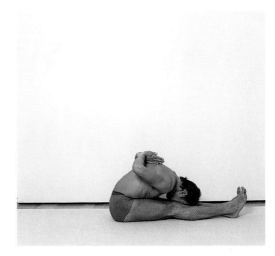

Inhaling, lift the hands off the floor and clasp them behind the back. Stretch and straighten the arms, open the chest, and expand the ribs. Exhaling, extend forward along the outstretched legs, drawing the chin toward the shins. Focusing on the resonance and rhythm of the breath, raise the arms up and over, toward the head. Close the chin upon the chest and direct the eyes toward the nose. Inhaling, release the hands and sit up. (See also Pure and Simple on page 79.)

Exhaling, sitting up straight and strong, take back the hands, extending the arms so that only the tips of the fingers touch the floor. Inhaling, roll back and press the whole of both of the hands into the ground. Simultaneously, lift the legs and buttocks away from the floor. Take the head back and draw the focus of the eyes to the center of the forehead. Drawing in the sacrum, push the feet to the floor right through to the tips of the toes. Paying attention to the smoothness and impact of the breath, increase the opening of the chest and the expansion of the ribcage. Exhaling, return to an upright position.

Inhaling, lift and open the arms to shoulder height. Exhaling, sweep the arms back and down, away from the body. As the fingers meet, bend the elbows and begin to draw the hands up the spine, pressing together the palms to form the reverse prayer position. Exhaling, extend forward, encouraging the chin to move toward the shins. Look down and in to the tip of the nose. Try to keep the elbows lifting and the palms pressing against each other. Extend the backs of the legs and grip the floor evenly. Inhaling, release the arm lock and return to an upright position.

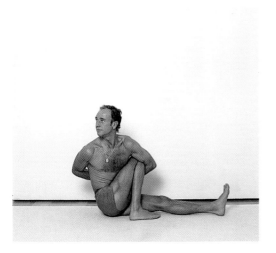
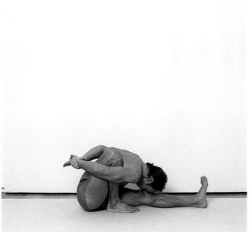
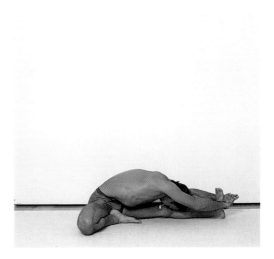

Exhaling, bend the right leg, taking the heel as close to the buttock as possible. Inhaling, turn to the right and simultaneously sweep the right arm around the back and the left arm over the right knee and back so the hands meet at the center of the spine. Tightly clasp the right hand over the left to promote a lift in the spine and an opening of the chest. Breathing deeply and evenly, rotate the head in the direction of the twist and bring the focal point to the corners of the eyes. Firmly press both the outstretched leg and the foot of the bent leg into the ground. Release the arm lock on an exhalation. Keep the bent leg in the same position and return to the center. (See also Pure and Simple on page 83.)

Inhaling, lift the chest and wrap the right arm around the right shin, taking the hand toward the spine. Carry the left arm back so the hands meet. Clasp the left wrist with the right hand and draw the spine in and up, keeping the chest and shoulders broad. Exhaling, extend the trunk forward and down, along the extending leg. Try to touch the shin with the chin and focus the eyes softly on the tip of the nose. Breathing deeply and rhythmically, pull the arms tight to increase the opening of the shoulders and broaden the back. The extending leg and foot of the bent leg maintain a strong connection with the floor. Release the arm lock on an inhalation and sit up, keeping the bent leg in the same position.

Exhaling, lower the right knee to the floor and turn the foot so the heel faces up and the bridge of the foot is flat on the floor. The angle between the right leg and the outstretched leg should be 120 degrees. Catch hold of the foot of the extending leg, breathe in, and draw the spine into the body. Exhaling, fold forward over the extending leg and tuck the chin to the chest. Focus the eyes on the tip of the nose. Breathing rhythmically and purposefully, continue to extend down the front of the outstretched leg. Drop the elbows toward the floor to ensure the back and shoulders broaden. Inhaling and keeping hold of the foot, raise the trunk. Exhaling, release the hands from the foot.

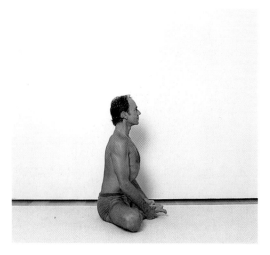
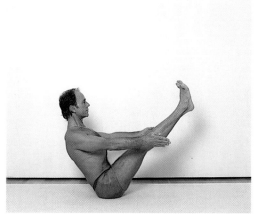

Inhaling, carry the left foot to meet the right and, taking hold of both feet with the hands, turn the soles of the feet, opening them like a book. Keep the outer edges of the feet together and the knees drawn down to the ground. Breathing freely and evenly, pull the feet as close to the perineum as possible, so the pelvis tilts forward. Move the sacrum and lower back inward and draw the upper spine in and up. The activity of the arms opens the shoulders and chest, increasing the life of the posture. Keep the abdomen long and hollow, the trunk elevated, and gaze into the mid-distance. Exhaling, release the hands from the feet.

Inhaling, place the hands on the floor and, taking the feet off the floor, bring the knees together. On an exhalation, extend the feet and legs upward, bringing them to head height. Lift the hands and arms forward, straight and in line with the shoulders. Balance on the sitting bones, breathe deeply and rhythmically, and pay attention to lifting the spine and chest. Keep the arms rigid and stretch evenly through the four corners of the wrist, the palms, and along to the fingertips. Continue to focus the eyes into the mid-distance. Exhaling, release from the posture, bending the legs and taking the hands to the floor at the side of the hips. Lift the buttocks and feet and sweep the legs through the hands back into Dog Pose.

Repeat the sequence, exchanging left for right and vice versa.
This completes one cycle of Sitting sequence III.

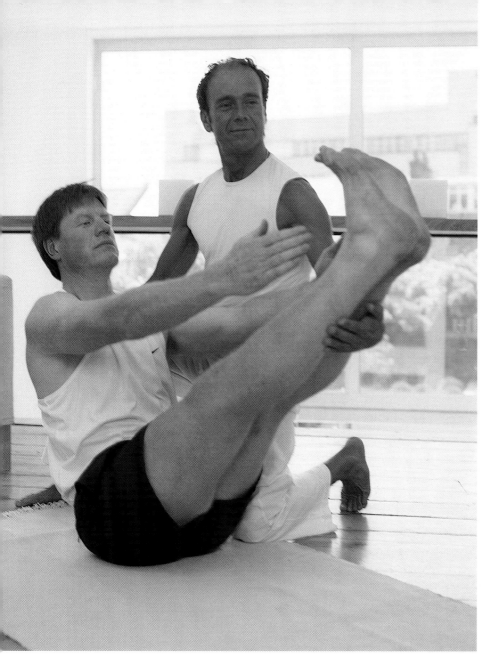

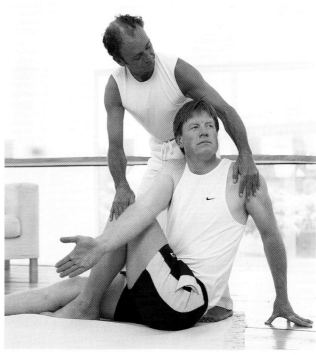

PURE AND SIMPLE

• ROTATING THE TRUNK AND SPINE EXERTS A STRONG INFLUENCE UPON THE VITAL ORGANS OF THE BODY. THE PRESSURE OF THE THIGH AGAINST ONE SIDE OF THE ABDOMEN AND CHEST STIMULATES BLOOD FLOW, TONING AND ERADICATING SLUGGISHNESS OF THE LIVER AND SPLEEN.

• THE HIPS AND SHOULDERS REGAIN THEIR NATURAL MOBILITY, AND TENSION IN THE NECK IS RELEASED.

• SEE ALSO POSTURE 5 ON PAGE 81.

We must realize from the outset that the legs

and arms are simply the instruments used to

enliven and stimulate the entire body/mind.

Inverted sequences

Altered states

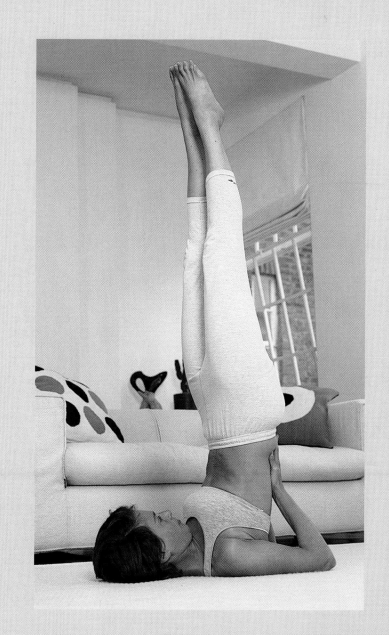

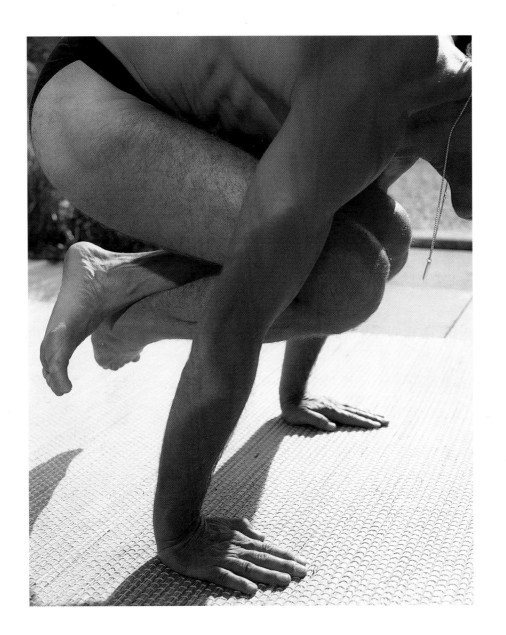

The inverted postures are generally the most powerful and offer the greatest benefits and rewards; they are therefore often the most challenging. This is because they literally turn our world upside-down. As human beings, we live and cope with the force of gravity. Evolution has transformed us into erect, upright individuals who are accustomed to the 15 pounds-per-square-inch that the gravitational pull exerts upon us. As such, our muscles, joints, and bones have the innate and natural ability to lift, support, and carry us. The practice of the Standing sequences deepens this ability and reinstructs us in the art of deportment and good carriage. However, by turning the body upside-down, there is a significant and powerful increase in the effects of gravity upon the entire body.

The musculo-skeletal systems are ordered and instructed to lift and support each other in the opposite direction to their customary way. This has the effect of dramatically strengthening the body and, upon returning to an upright position, the force and effect of gravity is mitigated. The intelligence of this series of postures is further revealed by the impact they have on all the bio-energy systems of the body. The reversal of the usual proximity of organs' tissue upon each other enlivens and refreshes them, and encourages the release of toxins and waste matter. Venous blood flows freely to the heart with the assistance of gravity, rather than against it. This activity strengthens the heart muscle, thereby improving the functioning of the circulatory system. The placement of the chin against the chest produces a lock that filters and regulates blood flow through the thyroid and para-thyroid glands into the brain. This has a decisive effect on the endocrine glands and nervous system, as not only is the brain soothed and softened, but also the metabolic rate of the body is regulated.

With practice, inverting the body encourages and aids natural, deep breathing by opening the upper lungs and ribs. However, at first, breathing may be difficult and restricted, which is why it is advisable to practice and master the first sequence before attempting the second or third.

Inverted sequence I

The structure of this sequence is designed not only as a means to introduce the body to the inverted postures, but it is also a most effective tonic and exercise in its own right. Referring to the importance and influence of moving with the breath, this sequence echoes the actions and principles established in the Sun sequences. There is an even greater need to pay strict attention to the exact synchronization of each movement and breath, as the demands made by each separate action upon the respiratory system are increased. The initial lift of the body from the floor illustrates this (see Posture 2), as does the second, which requires control, concentration, and confidence to slowly and accurately lower the feet to the floor (see Posture 6).

Fluency only comes from repetition, and repetition ensures that the effects are implanted on a cellular level. Regular practice allied to precision and discipline turns gross, clumsy actions into refined, graceful, purposeful movements.

Because of the placement of the head, it is imperative that it is not turned or deflected in any way while moving from posture to posture. At times, the shoulders and neck support the entire weight of the body, so any minor displacement of the head and neck must be avoided. The neck and shoulders are refreshed, and the pressure of the chin-lock is released by the maintenance of the penultimate posture (Posture 8). This ensures and promotes a balancing effect upon the neck, and stimulates blood circulation to the brain. From the fullness of the process, muscle tone is enhanced, organ tissue is stimulated, and consequently energy levels soar.

PURE AND SIMPLE ▶

• THE ENTIRE BODY LIFTS PERPENDICULAR TO THE FLOOR FROM THE IMPACT GENERATED BY THE DELIVERY OF AN INHALATION.

• THE MUSCLES OF THE BACK OF THE TRUNK AND THE ARMS HELP THE ELEVATION, AND THE STRONG GRIP OF THE LEG AND ABDOMINAL MUSCLES PROMOTE ACCURATE ALIGNMENT.

• SEE ALSO POSTURE 2, OVERLEAF.

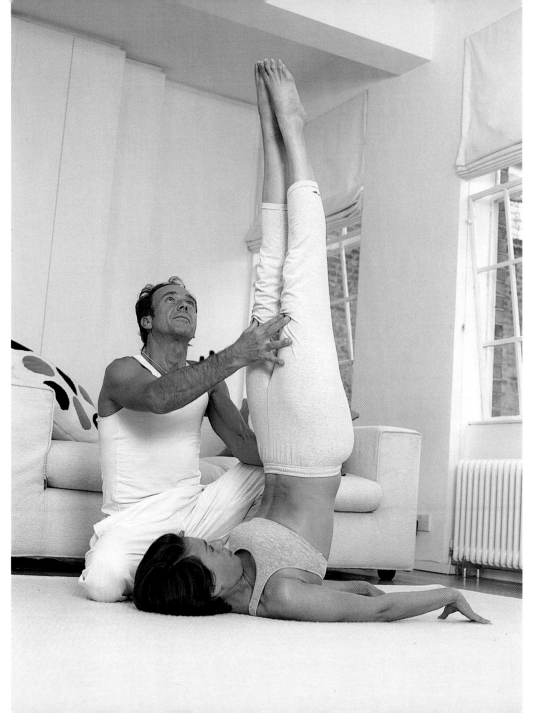

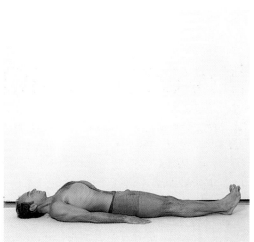

1 Lying flat on the floor and **exhaling,** stretch the body evenly and equally. Extending the legs away from the spine and lengthening the arms, push the palms of the hands firmly into the floor at the sides of the hips or thighs. The chest is broad, the abdomen long and hollow. The back of the neck is stretched. Look up toward the sky, focusing on the mid-distance.

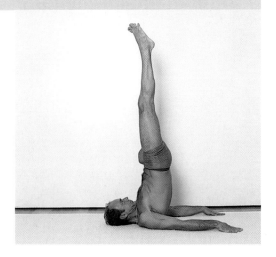
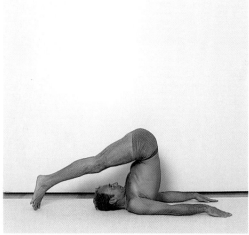
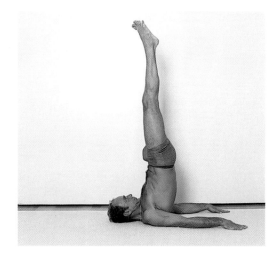

2 Inhaling deeply and powerfully, lift the feet, legs, and trunk up high so that the whole body comes to a vertical position. Keep the arms fixed to the floor with the wrists pushing firmly into the ground. Draw the spine into the body and increase this extension all the way through the legs, right to the tips of the toes. Nestle the chest against the chin and look toward the navel. (See also Pure and Simple on page 88.)

3 Exhaling and keeping the arms active and strong, begin to lower the feet and legs to the floor behind the head. The spine remains lifted and the legs are active and stretched. As the feet touch the floor tuck in the sacrum and contract the lower abdomen to its fullest. Keep the chest touching the chin and focus on the navel. (See also Pure and Simple on page 93.)

4 Inhaling, lift the legs and feet straight back up to a vertical position. The lift is supplied by the strong grip of the abdominal and back muscles and the bracing action of the arms. Keep the legs active and stretch the feet up to the sky. Focus on the navel and keep the chin in contact with the chest.

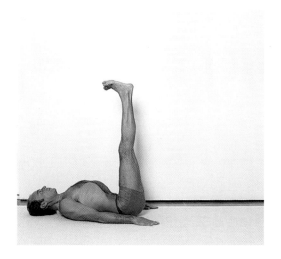 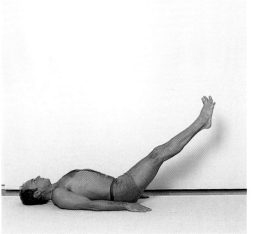 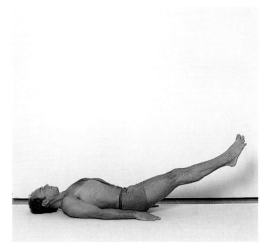

5 **Exhaling** and keeping the legs rigid and firm, carefully lower the whole spine and trunk to the floor. Pay attention to the quality of the breath as the vertebrae meet the ground sequentially. The chest broadens, the abdomen lengthens, and, as the sacrum touches the floor, the lumbar vertebrae lift up and away from the ground. The legs are vertical. Focus on the toes.

6 **Inhaling,** slowly lower the feet and legs toward the floor, maintaining the lift of the lumbar spine and activity throughout the arms. The chest broadens and opens, the abdomen lengthens, and the diaphragm stays soft. At the end of the inhalation, suspend the feet away from the floor. Focus on the mid-distance.

7 **Exhaling,** tightly grip together the inner edges of the feet and legs, keeping the feet suspended off the floor. Draw the lumbar vertebrae deeper into the body, brace the arm muscles more firmly, and increase the grip of the intercostal muscles upon the lower ribs. Keep the chest and shoulders broad throughout. Lock the lower abdomen to support the legs, and maintain the focus of the eyes on the mid-distance.

Repeat Postures 1 to 7 six to eight times (according to capacity) before moving into the next posture.

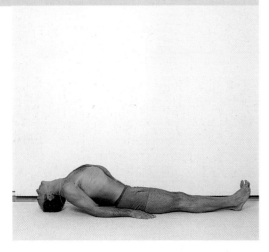

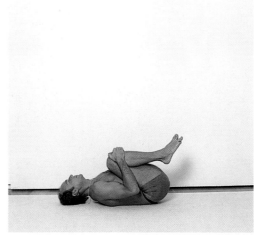

8 **Inhaling** and lying flat on the floor, arch the whole back and rest the crown of the head on the floor. Look up and in to the center of the brow, and stretch the front of the neck to its maximum. Breathing evenly and deeply, pay attention to the strong supportive action of the arms and the legs. Apply downward pressure to increase the upward lift of the chest and spine. Lengthen the abdomen and keep the diaphragm soft and open. (See also Pure and Simple, opposite.)

9 **Exhaling,** lie back down, taking the spine to the floor and the knees to the chest. Catch hold of the shins or ankles with the hands and flex the spine by gently rocking and rolling from side to side and backward and forward. Breathing rhythmically and evenly, keep the back of the head on the floor, and direct the focus of the eyes to the tip of the nose.

This completes one cycle of Inverted sequence I.

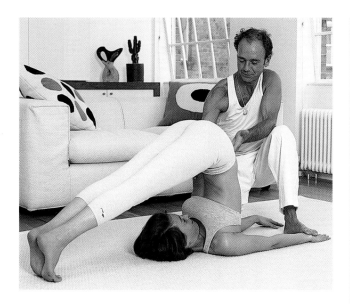

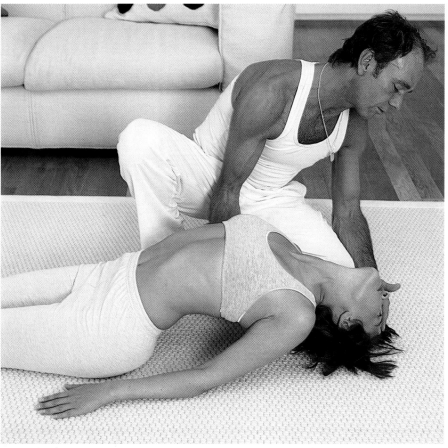

▲ PURE AND SIMPLE

• THE ARMS EXTEND OUT OF THE SHOULDER GIRDLE AND
ANCHOR THE POSTURE. THE SPINE DRAWS IN AND UP
AND THE LEGS REMAIN RIGID, STRONG, AND FIRM
THROUGHOUT THE MOVEMENT. THE FEET SHOULD MEET
THE FLOOR SILENTLY.

• SEE ALSO POSTURE 3 ON PAGE 90.

▲ PURE AND SIMPLE

• IN THIS POSTURE, THE CHEST IS WELL EXPANDED AND AS THE DIAPHRAGM IS OPEN AND STRETCHED,
BREATHING BECOMES FULLER AND EASIER.

• THE OPENNESS OF THE CHEST IS CARRIED THROUGH TO THE NECK, WHICH STIMULATES THE THYROID
GLANDS AND COUNTER-POSES THE CONTRACTION OF THE WINDPIPE AND THROAT.

• SEE ALSO POSTURE 8, OPPOSITE.

Inverted sequence II

The range of postures is broader and calmer in this sequence, and the first three postures are held and maintained for an increasing amount of time as practice develops. With inner attention and awareness, the mind is given the opportunity to fine-tune the subtle actions of the body and to refine the mechanics of the respiratory system. These postures provide the perfect environment for awakening and developing the inner organs of perception. Sustaining these primary postures breeds stamina, strength, and intimacy.

    The following variations are devices that both task and educate the individual muscle groups and skeletal frame. Alternating between extension and lift, the legs are used to liberate and tone the spine and abdominal wall equally. The activity of the arms is no less important than the legs, as they are used to either support, direct, or increase extension and awareness. As with the first sequence, the final posture of this series balances the others through the medium of contrast. The degree of difficulty of the posture is increased by the suspension of the feet and legs further from the floor. The thorough and diverse stimulation of the whole of the body produces a self-sufficiency and calm authority, which is a rare commodity today.

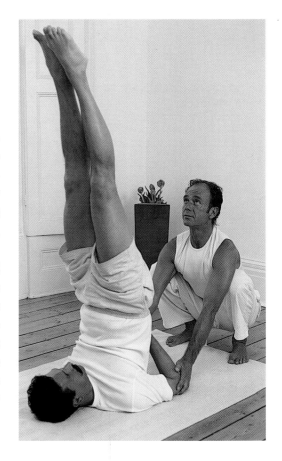

PURE AND SIMPLE

• THE PALMS ARE KEPT IN LINE WITH THE WRISTS AND FOREARMS.

• THE ELBOWS DRAW TOWARD EACH OTHER, OPENING THE SHOULDER GIRDLE AND DEVELOPING THE MUSCLES OF THE UPPER ARM.

• THE STABILITY AND LIFE OF THE POSTURE IS INITIATED BY THIS ACTION AND IS THEN TRANSLATED THROUGH TO THE TRUNK AND LEGS.

• SEE ALSO POSTURE 2, OPPOSITE.

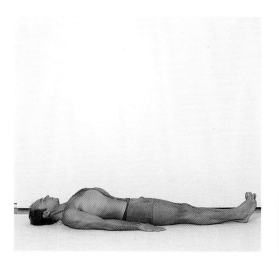

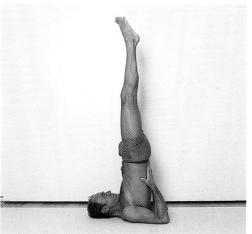

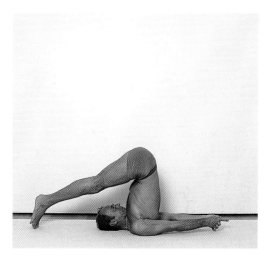

1 **Exhaling,** lie down flat, extending the legs away and out of the hip sockets, and pressing the heels firmly into the floor. Extend the arms, lengthening through to the fingers. Push the palms of the hands into the ground. Broaden the chest and shoulders, keep the abdomen long and hollow, and softly focus the eyes up to the open sky.

2 **Inhaling,** raise the trunk and legs so the entire body is perpendicular. Exhaling, bend the arms at the elbows and draw the palms to either side of the spine. Breathing fully and evenly, check the palms of the hands and the forearms are on the same line. The wrists should not twist or collapse. Draw the entire spine in and up, marrying the action of the lower abdomen with that of the lower back. Actively extend the legs upward, brace the inner knees apart, and tightly grip the feet together. Focus the gaze on the navel and keep the chin firmly pressed against the chest. Pay attention to the resonance and smoothness of the breath. (See also Pure and Simple, opposite.)

3 **Exhaling slowly and carefully,** lower the feet and legs behind the head to the floor. Keep the legs straight throughout this movement. As the feet touch the floor, simultaneously lock the lower abdomen and draw in the sacrum, maintaining a straight and natural spine. Breathing deeply and evenly, interlock the fingers and straighten the arms, taking the clasped hands to the floor. Keep looking at the navel.

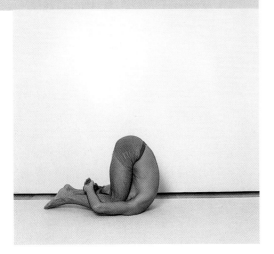 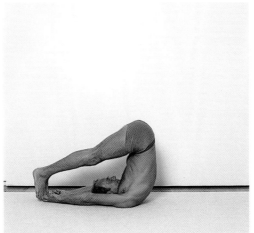 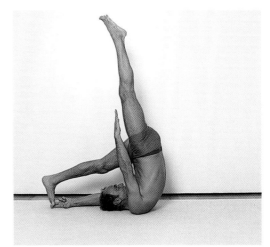

4 **Exhaling,** bend and lower the knees toward the ears, taking the bridges of the feet to the floor. Release the interlocked hands and carry them over to the legs, resting the forearms on the backs of the calves. Move the focus of the eyes to the tip of the nose and continue breathing in a considered and deliberate manner. Stretch the back of the body and compress the chest and abdomen.

5 **Inhaling,** stretch and straighten the arms and legs, taking the hands to the feet. Using the grip of the arms and legs to increase the traction of the spine, draw the trunk in and up. Breathing rhythmically and smoothly, push up the hips and tailbone and draw in the sacrum. Lock the lower abdomen and lengthen the trunk. Focus the gaze on the navel.

6 **Inhaling,** raise the right arm and leg simultaneously. The arm follows the leg with the outstretched hand pointing to the extending toes. The action of both legs is strong and even. Maintain the focus on the navel and, on an exhalation, return the arm and leg to the floor. Repeat the action to the other side. After three repetitions, breathing rhythmically and evenly, take the feet and hands back to the floor behind the head, as in Posture 5. (See also Pure and Simple on page 99.)

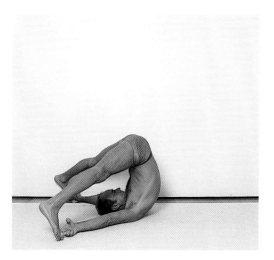

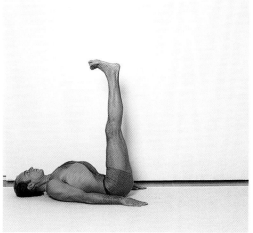

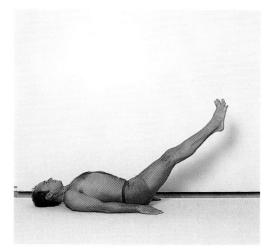

7 **Inhaling,** carry both feet and arms as wide as possible, maintaining the lift of the spine. Stretch the legs fully and evenly, employing them to lengthen the trunk, broaden the shoulders, and open the hips. Pay attention to the quality of each and every breath, and increase the opening of the chest. Focus on the navel.

8 **Exhaling,** draw together the feet, legs, and hands and, after releasing the feet from the hands, slowly lower the back and trunk to the floor. Next, take the arms up and over so they lie at the sides of the trunk.

9 **Inhaling,** slowly and methodically lower the straight legs down to the floor. Watch carefully that the movement does not become jerky or quick as this reveals a lack of control or concentration. Concentrating on the smoothness of the breath and the strength and life of the legs ensures that the movement is both elegant and purposeful. At the summit of the inhalation, the heels gently meet the floor so the whole body now lies flat and out-stretched.

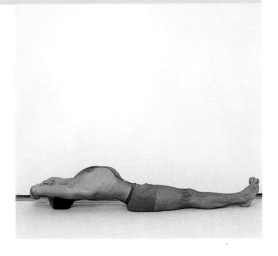

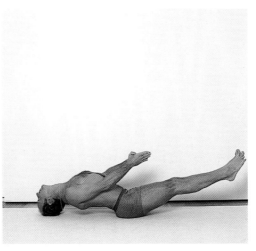

PURE AND SIMPLE ▶
• LOCKING THE FEET AND LEGS TOGETHER INCREASES THE ACTIVITY AND INTEGRITY OF ACTION OF THE LOWER ABDOMINAL WALL. THE CONSCIOUS EXTENSION OF THE ARMS, THROUGH TO THE FINGERS AND HANDS, MAINTAINS THE OPENING OF THE CHEST AND SHOULDERS. IT IS FROM THESE TWO SIMILAR ACTIONS THAT SPACE IS PROVIDED FOR THE SPINE TO LIFT AND DRAW INTO THE BODY.
• SEE ALSO POSTURE 6 ON PAGE 96.

10 **Inhaling,** arch the spine and neck, coming to rest on the crown of the head. On the same breath, lift the arms up and over the head. Bending the elbows, take the right hand to the left elbow and the left hand to the right elbow, encouraging the weight of the arms to increase both the lift of the spine and the opening of the chest. Breathing deeply and rhythmically, turn the focus of the eyes to the center of the brow. Anchor the posture with the legs and extend out of the hips, pressing firmly into the floor. Lengthen the abdomen and broaden the diaphragm so it is open and soft.

11 **Exhaling,** release the arm-lock and take the arms and hands forward, bringing the palms together to form the prayer position. At the same time, raise the feet off the floor so the arms and legs are on the same plane. Maintaining awareness of the quality of each breath, keep focusing upon the center of the brow. Exhaling, release from the posture and lie down flat. (See also Pure and Simple, opposite.)

This completes one cycle of Inverted sequence II.

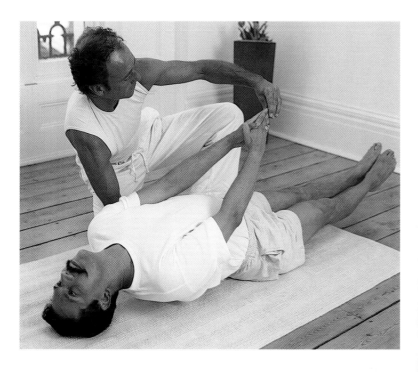

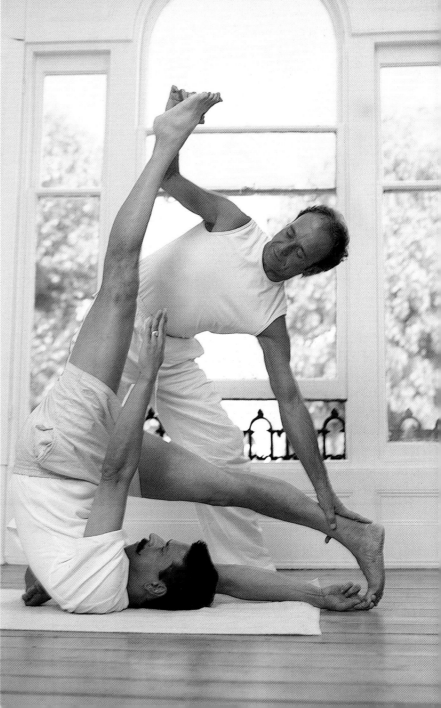

PURE AND SIMPLE ▶

• THE EVEN AND COMPLETE EXTENSION OF BOTH ARMS AND LEGS IS
ONLY POSSIBLE BY PAYING CLOSE AND CAREFUL ATTENTION TO THE
SYNCHRONIZATION OF EACH MOVEMENT WITH EACH BREATH.
• THIS ENSURES NOT ONLY RAPID, SAFE PROGRESS BUT ALSO ESTABLISHES
AN IMPLICIT QUALITY OF PRACTICE.
• SEE ALSO POSTURE 11, LEFT.

Inverted sequence III

Too often we consider the postures to be of paramount importance, and in our ambition to create a certain shape or form, we disregard the *modus operandi*. Each movement and posture of this sequence necessitates deliberate, acute concentration, and it is only this attitude that coerces the body to open and release naturally and voluntarily. As the emphasis of this sequence is rooted in the techniques of opening and expanding the entire body to its fullest, pay particular attention to the accurate placement of the hands on the spine. Attending to this detail will relieve pressure from the wrists and instruct the spine to move deeper into the trunk.

The information gleaned from the initial actions of this sequence can be regarded as preparation for the practice of the final two postures. Unless we have a predisposition for back bending, these two postures can seem intimidating and unnerving. The dramatic opening of the heart center often reveals our latent fears and insecurity. So that we are able to face these fears, it is essential that each separate instruction and direction is applied and adhered to, since taking a methodical and considered approach provides composure and inner quiet. It is in the balance between the inner calm and application of the mind, with the resultant vitality and vigor of the body, that the true benefits of practice begin to unfold.

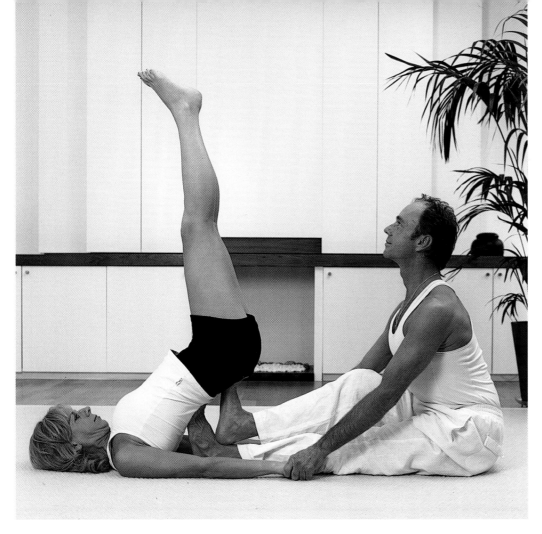

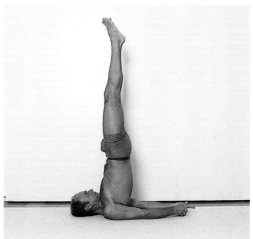

1 **Inhaling,** and lying flat, raise the whole body until it is perpendicular. Take the hands away from the trunk and tightly clasp the hands, lengthening the arms and broadening the shoulders. Keep the legs and arms strong and active. Brace apart the inner knees and, conversely, press together the inner edges of the feet. Breathing fully and evenly, draw in the sacrum and lock the lower abdomen so the trunk lengthens, opening and softening the diaphragm. Gently focus the eyes on the navel.

PURE AND SIMPLE

• THE RELEASE OF THE LOWER BACK AND SPINE REMOVES TENSION FROM THE NECK AND SHOULDERS AND ESTABLISHES THE ESSENTIAL ACTION NECESSARY FOR THE UPPER SPINE TO LIFT AND THE CHEST TO BROADEN.

• SEE ALSO POSTURE 2, OVERLEAF.

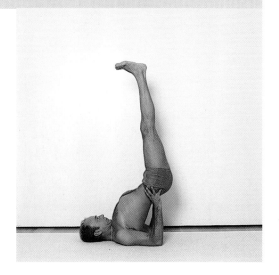 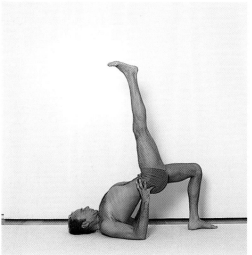 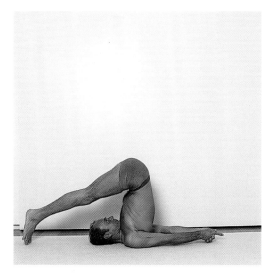

2 Exhaling, release the arm-lock and bend the elbows, taking the hands toward the spine. On the same breath, arch the back and lower the sacrum on to the palms of the hands. Continuing to breathe in a controlled and even manner, keep looking toward the navel. Drawing the spine into the body relieves pressure in the wrists and increases the opening of the chest and lungs. Keep the legs active and lifted, away from the gravitational pull. (See also Pure and Simple on page 101.)

3 Inhaling, bend and lower the left leg over the hands to the floor. Make this action considered and deliberate, resisting the temptation to drop the foot to the floor. Deepen the lift and arch of the spine, increasing the stretch of the face of the body. Keep the upward leg firm and active. Hold the focus of the gaze upon the navel. Exhaling, raise the left leg and, on the following inhalation, repeat this action on the other side.

4 Exhaling, lower both legs straight back over the head, taking the arms and hands back to the floor. Keep the palms on either side of the spine. Ensure that the legs are active, straight, and strong, and the abdomen lengthened. Expand the whole of the back of the lungs and spine so they are stretched long and broad. Focus the eyes on the navel and firmly connect the chin and chest.

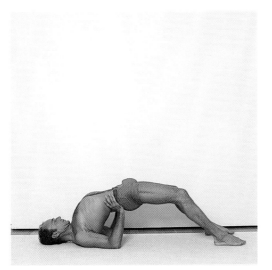 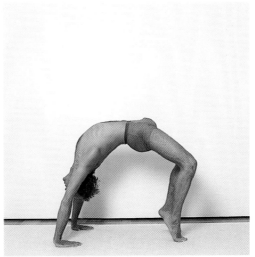 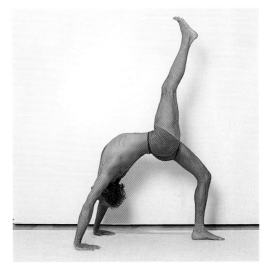

5 **Inhaling deeply,** take the hands back to the spine and then lift up both legs straight and, on the same breath, carry them over the hands to the floor, away from the head. Walk the feet away from the hands, straightening them as much as possible. Stretch evenly throughout the extending legs, drawing the sacrum and entire spine deep into the body. Keep the eyes focused in the direction of the navel and continue breathing rhythmically and purposefully. Stretch the abdomen and widen the diaphragm so the entire chest is expanded. (See also Pure and Simple on page 104.)

6 **Exhaling,** bend the knees, walking the feet back toward the hips and coming on to tiptoes. Maintaining the arch of the spine, release the hands and lift them up and over, placing the palms flat on the floor under the shoulders with the fingers pointing in the direction of the feet. Inhaling, roll on to the crown of the head and, pressing the palms and the flat of the toes into the floor, lift the body, arching the spine. Look to the center of the forehead, draw back the head between the shoulders, and extend the chest and abdomen to their maximum. Breathing as freely and deeply as possible, pay attention to the equality of action between the hands and feet, and the legs and arms.

7 **Exhaling,** press the left foot flat into the floor, bend the right knee, and take the thigh to meet the chest. Focus carefully on the action and activity of the supporting leg, and the strength delivered by the hands and arms. On an inhalation, elevate the upper leg so the toes stretch up to the sky. The lower abdomen contracts deeply, the abdominal wall is taut, and the chest and lungs expand to their fullest. Hold the gaze point at the center of the brow. Repeat this action to the other side. (See also Pure and Simple on page 105.)

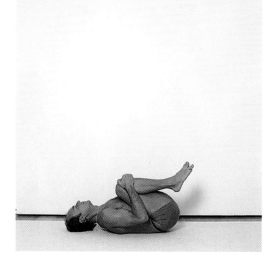

8 **Exhaling,** release and lie down flat on the floor. Bend the knees and bring both thighs to the chest. Catch the ankles or shins and pull the legs against the abdomen and chest. Rest the back of the head on the floor and rock sensitively, backward and forward, and side to side, giving the spine a gentle massage. Breathing deeply and evenly, gaze softly into the mid-distance.

This completes one cycle of Inverted sequence III.

▼ PURE AND SIMPLE

• DETERMINED APPLICATION IS REQUIRED TO ENCOURAGE THE LEGS TO STRAIGHTEN AND LENGTHEN, THE TOES STRETCH OUT, AND THE FEET GRIP THE FLOOR.

• PRESSURE ON THE WRISTS AND ELBOWS IS LESSENED BY THE DUAL ACTION OF THE FEET PUSHING DOWN AND STRETCHING THE SPINE TOWARD THE NECK.

• SEE ALSO POSTURE 5 ON PAGE 103.

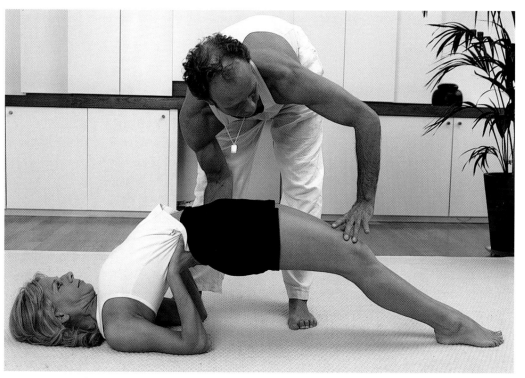

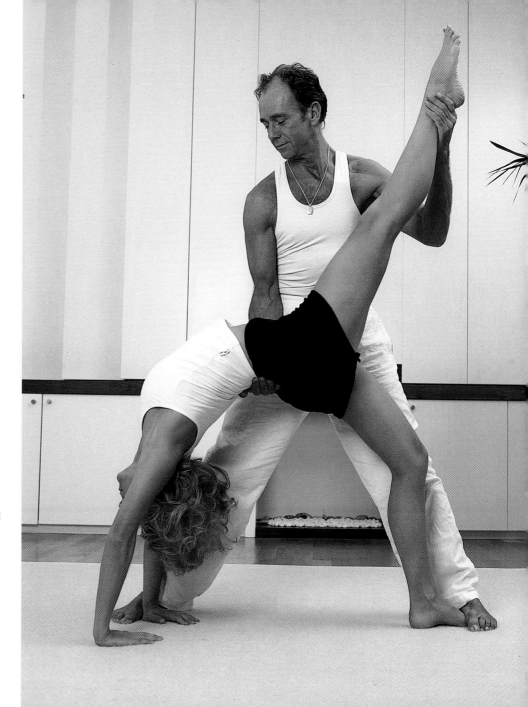

PURE AND SIMPLE

• THIS IS A WONDERFUL, EXPRESSIVE, AND AUTHORITATIVE
POSTURE. DESPITE THE ASYMMETRICAL FORM OF THIS
POSTURE, ITS EXECUTION DEMANDS AND PRODUCES
BALANCE AND EQUALITY OF ACTION.

• THE STRENGTH AND CONNECTION OF THE FOOT AND
HANDS WITH THE FLOOR IS IN EXACT PROPORTION TO
THE LIFE AND EXTENSION OF THE UPPER LEG.

• SEE ALSO POSTURE 7 ON PAGE 103.

It is in the balance between the inner calm and

application of the mind, with the resultant vitality

and vigor of the body, that the true benefits of

practice begin to unfold.

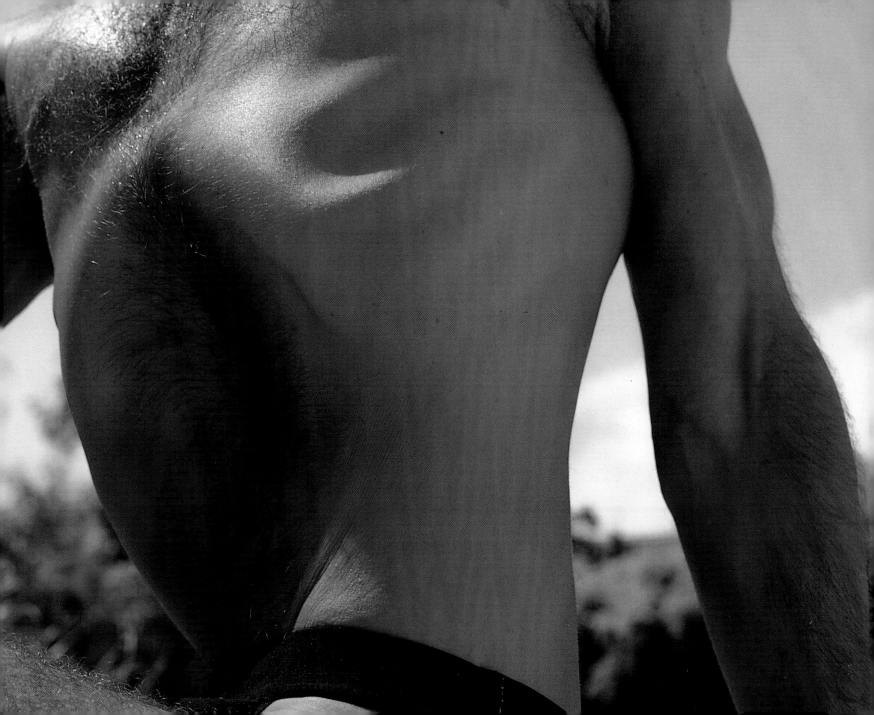

Supine sequences

Earthing and grounding

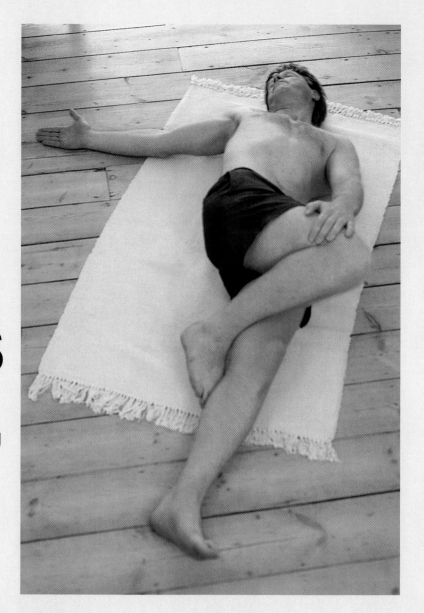

The impact of the inverted postures upon the body/mind is deep and profound, and therefore needs to be channeled deliberately and intelligently. The supine sequences offer an immediate antidote and complement to the stimulation of the nervous system and the increase of blood circulation.

Gravity is employed to sedate, soften, and soothe the nervous system in the following sequences, and to release any residual tension that may have been developed through assertive practice. The combination of the postures and movements with deep rhythmic breathing rejuvenates the body/mind and dispels lethargy and fatigue. As with every sequence, each and every action must be considered and controlled. The difference now is that the movements and postures are much simpler and ostensibly less demanding, though no less effective, than the previous sequences. This means that generally there is a greater opportunity for attention to detail, and attention to detail delivers the key to the door of refinement.

The majority of the postures in this chapter involve the spine and back of the ribcage being connected and pressed into the ground. This has the effect of both compressing the muscles of the back and restricting the expansion of the back of the ribcage. The face of the chest and frontal ribs are thus encouraged and directed to expand despite the restrictions imposed by the various extensions, rotations, and stretches that define the postures.

The previous sequences have been increasingly demanding and active. The opposite is true of this series of sequences. This is because their inherent quality is their ability to restore energy to the body/mind quietly and sensitively. Therefore, the progressive aspect of this series is directed toward developing the ability to consciously release tension and tightness, affording the opportunity to unwind. This skill is just as difficult as any other aspect of practice, but once acquired, escalates and elevates practice on to a different, higher plane.

Supine sequence I

In this, the first of the Supine sequences, considered actions are balanced with sustained extensions and stretches. The understanding gained from the practice of the previous sequences now proves to be invaluable as the need for control and concentration is heightened. The movements and positions at the beginning of the sequence, where the back of the lungs and spine are connected with the floor, mirror the actions of the inverted postures. From the influence made by natural, deep breathing the spine is encouraged to regain its natural form. A natural spine is curved, not straight. This means that the sacrum must press into the ground and the lumbar vertebrae must lift away from the ground to maintain and manufacture the natural form of the spine. The effects of this action guarantee a release of the diaphragm, restoring natural deep breathing. Continued and deepening awareness of this connective action should be made throughout every sequence. The last few postures of the series further this understanding and also increase the exchange of tension for release.

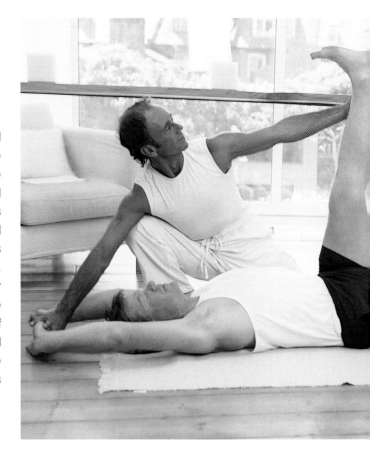

▲ **PURE AND SIMPLE**

• JUST AS MUCH ATTENTION AND ACTIVITY IS REQUIRED OF THE DOWNWARD LEG AS THE UPWARD, EXTENDING LEG.

• THE LENGTHENING AND STRETCH OF THE ARMS BACKWARD DEEPENS THE OPENING OF THE DIAPHRAGM AND INCREASES THE EXPANSION OF THE WHOLE OF THE CHEST AND LUNGS.

• SEE ALSO POSTURE 2, OPPOSITE.

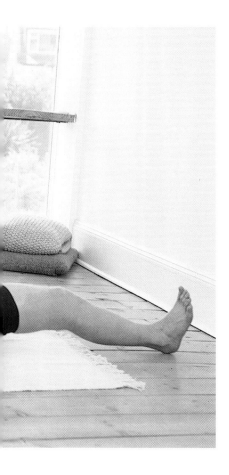

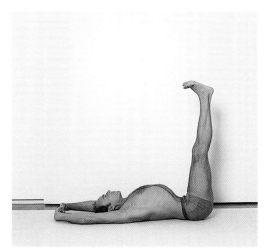

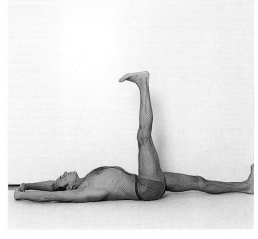

1 **Inhaling,** simultaneously raise the arms over the head to the floor and lift up both legs, keeping the sacrum and thoracic spine on the floor. Draw in the lumbar vertebrae, lock the lower abdomen, expand the chest, and soften and open the diaphragm. Breathing fully and evenly, tightly grip together the inner edges of the legs, stretching the backs of both legs and contracting the front of the thighs. Focus softly upon the toes and press the arms firmly into the floor.

2 **Exhaling,** lower the left leg to the floor, making sure the upward, lifting leg stays firm, straight, and strong. Keep the arms rooted to the floor and firmly press the heel of the downward leg into the ground. Remain focused on the upward, lifting leg, and breathe deeply and purposefully. Open the chest, lengthen the abdomen, and stretch the whole of the front of the trunk. Inhaling, raise the right leg. Repeat to the other side, alternating the action of the legs. (See also Pure and Simple, opposite.)

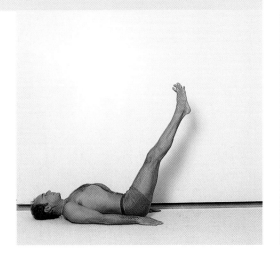

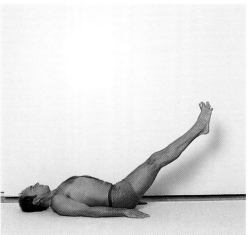

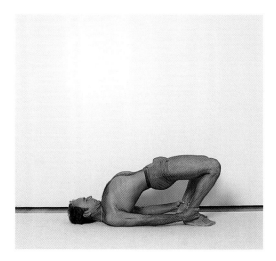

3 Exhaling and with strong legs, slowly lower the feet toward the floor. As they reach an angle of 60 degrees above the floor, hold them there. Take the arms down to the side of the trunk with palms facing down. Breathing as deeply and evenly as possible, focus on the mid-distance. Lift the lumbar spine deeper into the body, increasing the opening of the diaphragm and the expansion of the chest.

4 Exhaling, lower the legs until they are 30 degrees from the floor. Tightly grip together the feet and inner edges of the legs. Increase the life of the posture by paying careful attention to the quality and resonance of the breath. Continue to look into the mid-distance. Draw the lumbar vertebrae into the body, lengthening the trunk, softening the diaphragm, and increasing the expansion of the chest. Exhaling, lie down flat and draw the arms to the sides of the body, close to the thighs.

5 Inhaling, bend the knees and lift the feet off the floor, catching hold of the ankles or shins. Press the soles of the feet back into the floor, arch the back, and raise the chest to meet the chin. Tightly brace the arms and open the chest and shoulders, creating space for the spine to move into the body. Firmly push both feet into the ground. This action translates into the knees, broadening the pelvic girdle and opening the hips. Breathing deeply and resonantly, focus on the tip of the nose and draw awareness throughout the feet, legs, arms, and trunk. Stretch the diaphragm and lengthen the abdomen. (See also Pure and Simple on page 115.)

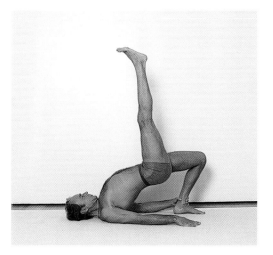

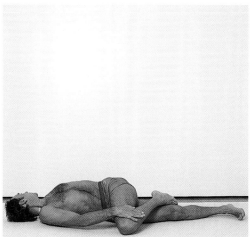

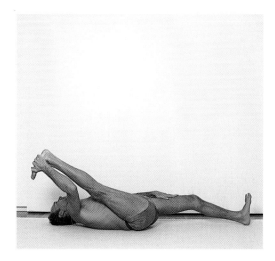

6 **Exhaling,** release the right hand from the right foot and raise the knee, taking the thigh to the chest. Inhaling, straighten the leg, pointing the foot up to the sky. The supporting foot and leg must now work harder to maintain the lift of the spine and the expansion of the chest. Deeply contract the lower abdomen to provide support for the elevated leg, which is firm and strong. Paying attention to the quality and impact of the breath, look at the toes of the extending foot. Repeat this action to the other side and then release from the posture on an exhalation, lying down flat.

7 **Inhaling,** carry the left arm wide, placing it flat on the floor, in line with the shoulders. At the same time, lift and bend the left leg at the knee, hooking the foot to the inside edge of the right thigh. Place the right hand on the left knee, encouraging the knee to move close to the floor, opening the hips, and broadening the sacroiliac. Keeping the neck long, turn the head to the left and focus on the tips of the fingers. Turn the palm face up and press the whole of the arm into the ground. Breathing freely and rhythmically, lengthen the abdomen and open the chest, drawing the spine into the body. Repeat this action to the other side and on an exhalation, lie flat on the floor.

8 **Exhaling,** bend and raise the right leg, catching the ankle or foot with both hands. On the same breath, begin to straighten the leg by bending the elbow and take the shin as close to the right ear as possible. Keeping the head on the floor, turn the gaze of the eyes to the toes of the upward leg. Deepening the stretch with each breath, draw awareness into the downward leg. Grip the floor with the back of the knee and extend evenly down through to the toes. Through the strong action of the arms, keep the spine and trunk long, the chest full and open, and the shoulders broad. Repeat the action with the left leg. Exhale and lie down flat on the floor.

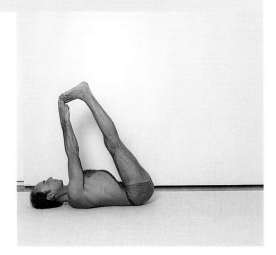

9 **Inhaling,** bend both knees and take hold of the front of the feet with both hands. Exhaling, begin to straighten arms and legs, maintaining contact between the sacrum and the floor. With equal force, pull down the arms and stretch up the legs. The activity of the arms broadens the chest and shoulders and the action of the legs broadens the hips and lower back. Focus on the feet and pay attention to the smoothness and resonance of the breath. Lengthen the abdomen and soften the diaphragm. Exhaling, release the feet and lie flat. (See also Pure and Simple, right.)

This completes one cycle of Supine sequence I.

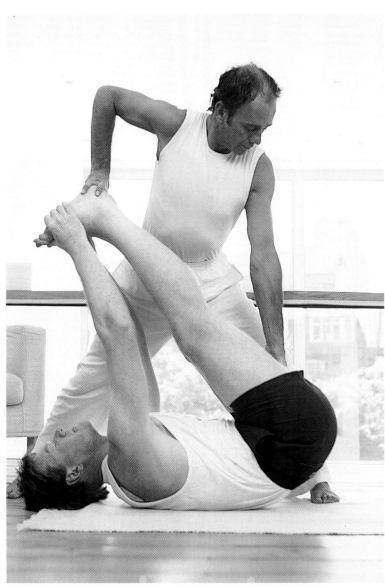

PURE AND SIMPLE

• THE FEET AND HANDS EXERT AN EQUAL PRESSURE UPON EACH OTHER.

• THE ARMS ARE LENGTHENED AND DRAW THE SHOULDERS DOWN TO THE GROUND, AND THE LEGS MIRROR THIS ACTION BY ENCOURAGING THE BASE OF THE SPINE TO MEET THE FLOOR.

• SEE ALSO POSTURE 9, LEFT.

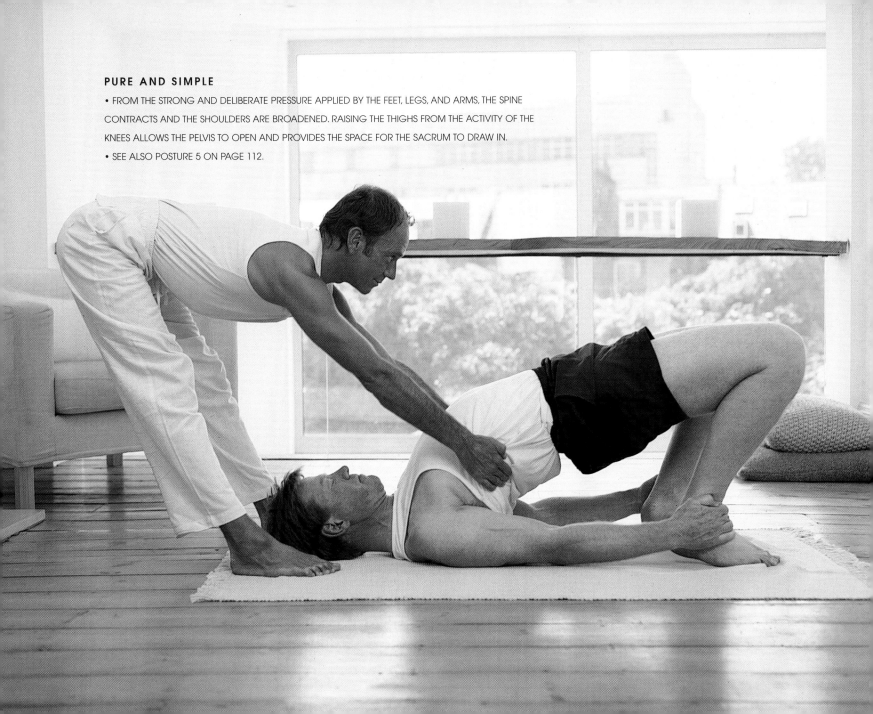

PURE AND SIMPLE

• FROM THE STRONG AND DELIBERATE PRESSURE APPLIED BY THE FEET, LEGS, AND ARMS, THE SPINE
CONTRACTS AND THE SHOULDERS ARE BROADENED. RAISING THE THIGHS FROM THE ACTIVITY OF THE
KNEES ALLOWS THE PELVIS TO OPEN AND PROVIDES THE SPACE FOR THE SACRUM TO DRAW IN.

• SEE ALSO POSTURE 5 ON PAGE 112.

Supine sequence II

Steadiness and precision are a prerequisite for this sequence. An increase in flexibility and integral awareness are the rewards. The maintenance of the postures provides space and time, allowing us to pay attention to the subtle actions and influence of the breath upon the body/mind. The arms and legs are used to express the hips and shoulders and to lengthen and tone muscle tissue. They also encourage the innate understanding of the connection and influence of the breath upon the body and of the posture on the breath. Adoption of this attitude rather than "stretching for the sake of stretch," increases the ability to locate areas of inactivity and to deepen the release of tension. Flowing, rhythmic breaths carry the arms and legs from posture to posture in sweeping movements. The postures both contrast and complement each other to further describe the respective target or essence of each posture. Beyond the physical benefits of an increase in blood flow and the release of tension, a calm, open, receptive quality of mind is developed. This results in an increase in intimate awareness, which has a profound and lasting effect upon the entire body/mind.

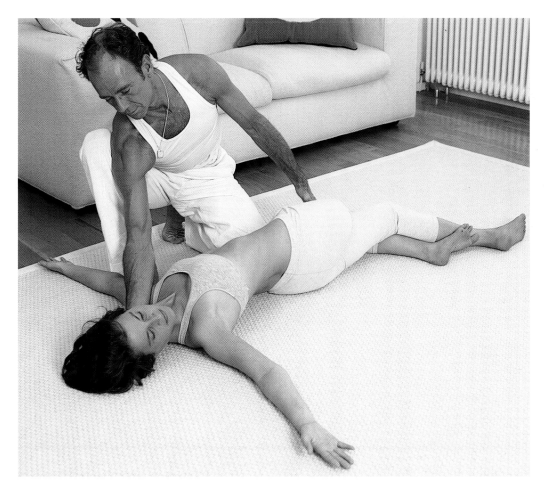

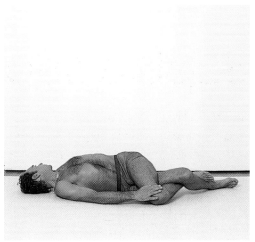

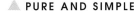

▲ PURE AND SIMPLE

• THE HEAD TURNS AWAY FROM THE ROTATING UPPER LEG AND HIP TO INCREASE THE STIMULUS OF THE SPINE.

• PRESSING THE ARMS INTO THE FLOOR PROVIDES STABILITY AND A BASE FROM WHICH THE SPINE CAN MOVE. GRIPPING THE FOOT AGAINST THE CALF INCREASES THE OPENING OF THE HIPS AND GROUNDS THE POSTURE.

• SEE ALSO POSTURE 1, RIGHT.

1 **Exhaling,** wrap the left leg over the right, taking the bridge of the left foot to the back of the right calf. Tightly grip together the legs and lower the left knee to the right-hand side of the body. Inhaling, sweep the left arm wide so it comes into line with the shoulders. At the same time, take the right hand to the left knee and turn the head to the right and focus on the fingers of the outstretched left hand. Breathing freely and rhythmically, increase the opening of the hips by lengthening the left leg as much as possible, encouraging the left knee to move closer to the floor. Twist and stretch the abdominal wall and draw in and rotate the spine. Exhaling, release the legs and lie back down flat. (See also Pure and Simple, left.)

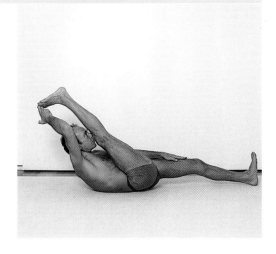
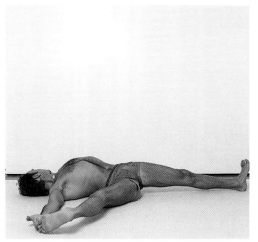
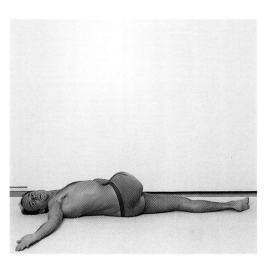

2 Inhaling, bend the right leg and catch hold of the neck of the big toe with the first two fingers of the right hand. Exhaling, begin to straighten the leg and, at the same time, bend the right elbow and take the chin toward the shin. Breathing deeply and resonantly, extend the left arm down the front of the left thigh, paying attention to the activity and equality of action of both legs. Look up to the right foot and ensure that the toe pulls on the fingers with as much authority as the fingers pull on the toe. Exhaling and keeping hold of the toe, lower the back and head to the floor. (See also Pure and Simple on page 121.)

3 Inhaling and maintaining the grip of the fingers on the neck of the big toe, carry the right leg wide and down toward the ground. Move up the left arm so that both arms are in line with the shoulders and turn the head to look across at the outstretched left hand. Press the heel of the left leg firmly into the floor and fan the toes wide, deepening the contact of the back of the knee with the floor. Both legs are straight, strong, and active. Breathing freely and evenly, encourage the right leg to move closer to the floor, paying attention to the anchoring effect of the arms, lower abdomen, and extended left leg.

4 Inhaling, release the right foot from the hand and, keeping it straight and strong, carry it over the trunk to the opposite hand. Catch the foot in the left hand and turn the head and gaze-point to the outstretched right hand and arm. Bring awareness into the deep contraction of the lower abdomen, increasing the opening and expression of the right hip. Breathing rhythmically and evenly, press the outside edge of the left leg into the floor and draw the spine into the body, lengthening the trunk and opening the chest. The arms are active and anchor the rotation of the spine.

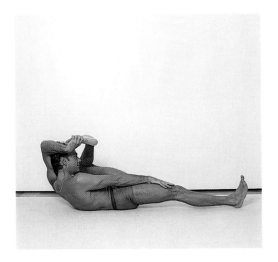
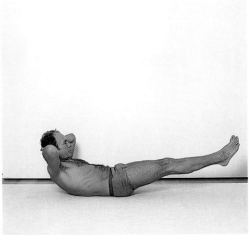
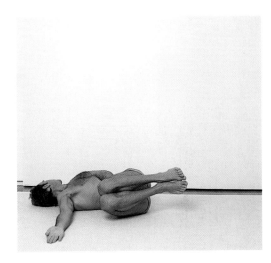

5 **Exhaling,** release the left foot and, centering the head, take the left hand around the base of the skull. Catch the outside edge of the left foot with the right hand and draw it to the left hand. Look to the tip of the nose and push back the head against the left arm. Extend the right hand along the front of the right thigh and brace the right leg into the ground. Paying attention to the resonance and quality of each breath, lock the lower abdomen and encourage the back to move to the floor. Exhaling, release and lie down flat. (See also Pure and Simple on page 120.)

Repeat Postures 1 to 5 to the other side, substituting right for left and vice versa.

6 **Inhaling,** take the palms to the back of the head. Exhaling, raise the head, trunk, and legs off the floor, maintaining the focus of the gaze on the tip of the nose. Draw the chin to the chest, move the elbows away from each other, and balance the whole body on the sacrum and lumbar vertebrae. Breathing as deeply and evenly as possible, tightly grip together the inner edges of the legs. Extend the legs evenly and equally, through to the tips of the toes. Deeply contract the lower abdomen and stretch the back of the ribcage and spine so the chest is full. Exhaling, release from the posture and lie down flat on the floor.

7 **Exhaling,** bend the knees and lift both legs up to the chest. At the same time, sweep the arms wide so they are in line with the shoulders. Exhaling, carry both legs over to the right elbow, turning the head and eyes to face the outstretched left hand. Suspend the knees and legs from the floor by the strong action of the lower abdominal wall and the contact made by the arms with the ground. Inhaling, raise the legs back up to the chest, turning the head back to the center. Repeat this action to the left-hand side and repeat the movements six to eight times, carefully synchronizing each movement with each breath. After the final repetition, with the knees close to the chest, exhale, take the hands to the ankles or shins.

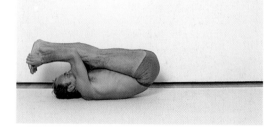

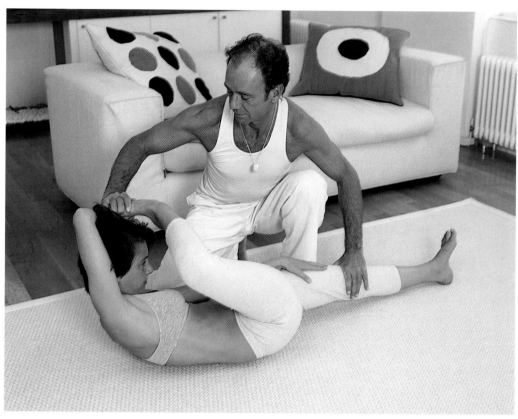

8 **Exhaling,** grip the hands on the sides of the feet and begin to straighten the legs. Broaden the elbows and pull the feet close to the head. Focus softly on the feet and hands and push the tailbone toward the ground. Pay attention to the depth and action of each breath, increasing the stretch of the legs to lengthen the spine. Lift the chest so it is open and broad, and brace the shoulders to provide space for the spine to draw into the body. Exhaling, release the hands and feet and lie flat on the floor.

This completes one cycle of Supine sequence II.

▲ **PURE AND SIMPLE**

• BRACING THE HEEL OF THE SUPPORTING LEG GENERATES STABILITY AND A FIRM GROUNDING OF THE LOWER SPINE.

• FROM THE STRENGTH SUPPLIED BY THE MUSCLES OF THE NECK THE BACK OF THE HEAD PUSHES AGAINST THE UPPER ARM INCREASING THE OPENING OF THE SHOULDERS AND HIPS. AS THIS IS BY FAR THE MOST COMPLICATED POSTURE OF THE SEQUENCE, EXTRA CARE AND ATTENTION MUST BE PLACED ON THE PRODUCTION OF EVEN, RHYTHMIC BREATHING.

• SEE ALSO POSTURE 5 ON PAGE 119.

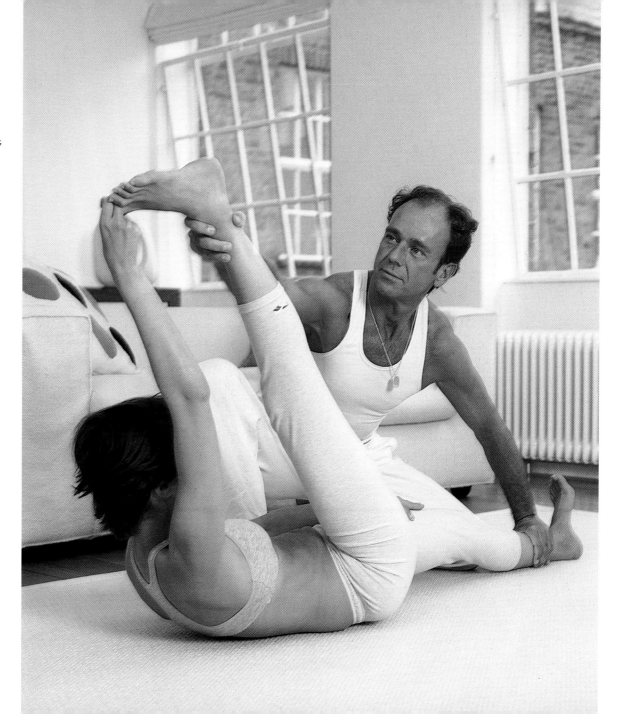

▶ **PURE AND SIMPLE**

MAINTAINING A FIRM CONTACT
BETWEEN THE FIRST TWO FINGERS AND
THE NECK OF THE BIG TOE OF THE LIFTING
FOOT ENSURES EQUALITY OF ACTION IN
THIS POSTURE.

• THE SHOULDERS AND HIPS RECEIVE
EQUAL ATTENTION, THE DOWNWARD
PRESSURE OF THE HEEL AND THE
EXTENSION OF THE LOWER ARM ENSURE
THAT BOTH SIDES OF THE BODY ARE
ACTIVE AND ALIVE.

• SEE ALSO POSTURE 2 ON PAGE 118.

Supine sequence III

This sequence is specifically designed to fit occasions when the body and mind no longer have the desire for further stimulus. Fatigue is never the sole province of the physical aspect of our being; when we are tired, it is often the case that the mind no longer seems to have the power to motivate the body. Creative self-expression becomes stifled, and the will-to-do dissolves. This program of postures restores and stimulates the body/mind with very little effort. The use of the wall to support the legs means that the postures almost do the work without any assistance or particular application. The only task we really need to undertake is to breathe as consciously and attentively as possible. If we apply our focus to the subtle mechanics of the respiratory system, the body will open, release, and realign itself. By giving the breath primacy, musculo-skeletal alignment is clarified by necessity. As the length of time spent in each posture increases, the legs and the trunk relinquish their weight to the gravity of the earth. The nervous system is thus soothed and softened, and deeply held latent tensions are absorbed into the ground from the body.

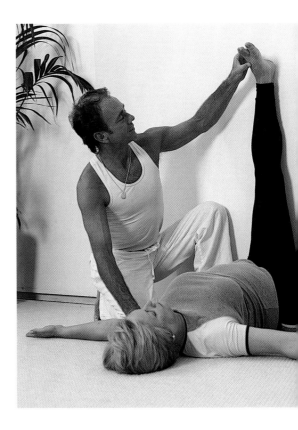

▲ PURE AND SIMPLE

• FROM THE LIFE AND LIFT OF THE UPPER LEG, THE EXTENDING LEG DRAWS CLOSER TO THE FLOOR AIDED BY GRAVITY. THE EXPANSION OF THE LUNGS AND THE OPENNESS OF THE CHEST ARE MAINTAINED BY THE STRETCH OF THE ARMS.

• SEE ALSO POSTURE 3 ON PAGE 124.

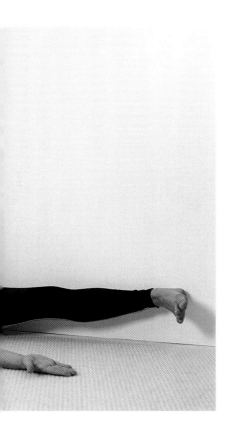

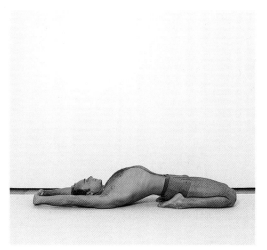

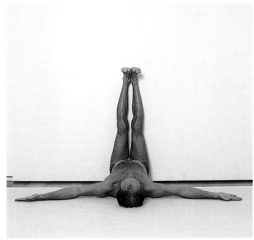

1 Kneel on the floor with the knees together and the buttocks flat on the floor. Place the feet at the sides of the hips and tuck in the calves to the back of the thighs. Breathing freely and resonantly, extend back and rest the elbows on the floor. Gradually lower the head and trunk down to the floor. **Inhaling,** sweep the arms up and back and clasp the hands, straightening the arms. Pull the sacrum into the body and brace the bridges of the feet into the ground. Expand the whole of the chest wall, lengthen the abdomen and trunk, and stretch the diaphragm wide and open. Exhaling, release from the posture and roll over to the right.

2 With the knees bent and over to one side, take the buttocks and feet as close to the wall as possible, centering the trunk and spine. **Exhaling,** raise the legs, pressing the backs of the legs flat against the wall. Point the toes and keep the legs active and strong. Inhaling, sweep the arms wide and lift the lumbar vertebrae away from the floor. Close the eyes and pay careful attention to the rhythm and impact of the breath upon the body. Follow the movement of the lungs, ribs, and spine, and the passage of the breath through the body.

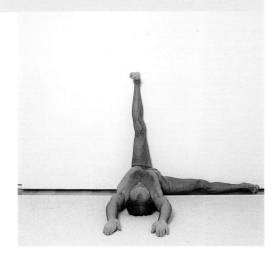

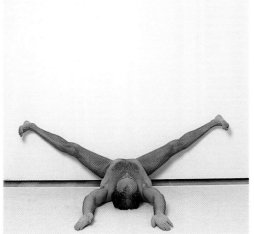

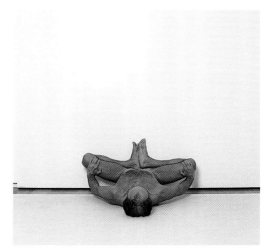

3 **Inhaling,** move the arms above the head. Keeping the eyes closed and the mind receptive and open, lower the right leg away from the left. Fix the mind's eye on the activity and stability of the left leg, as it is from the support provided by the upper leg that the lower leg extends. Maintain an even stretch throughout the arms and allow the force of gravity to increase the extension of the lower leg. Breathe in a more deep, controlled, and sensitive way. Gently raise the right leg and repeat for an equal amount of time to the other side. (See also Pure and Simple on page 122.)

4 Keeping the arms stretched back and **inhaling,** slowly spread the legs wide, lowering the feet down the wall. Keep activity in both legs, paying equal attention to the stretch of the outer thighs, knees, and feet and the inner knees, groin, and ankles. The lifting action of the lumbar vertebrae promotes a greater extension of the hips and groin and also increases the aperture of the diaphragm. Draw the mind into the sensations of stretch, lift, support, and release—not away from them.

5 With great sensitivity, **exhale** and begin to bend the knees. Maintaining the contact of the feet with the wall, draw the feet toward each other. As they meet, press together the soles of the feet and take them as low down the wall as possible. With the heels close to the root of the groin, take the hands to the knees and begin to apply mild pressure, encouraging the knees to move to the wall. Gauge the degree of resistance in the groin against the ability to soften and release tension, gradually dissolving tension through the direct application of concentrated awareness. Exhaling, quietly roll out of the posture, open the eyes, and come into enough space to lie down flat. (See also Pure and Simple, opposite.)

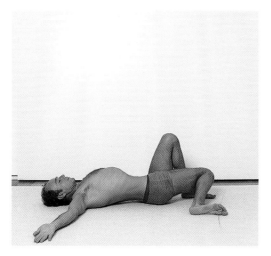

▼ **PURE AND SIMPLE**

• ONLY MILD PRESSURE IS APPLIED TO THE KNEES BY THE HANDS. THE GROIN CAN BE STUBBORN AND RESISTANT, AND DEMAND SENSITIVITY AND UNDERSTANDING BEFORE IT WILL SUBMIT TO THE COMMANDS OF THE MIND.

• SEE ALSO POSTURE 5, OPPOSITE.

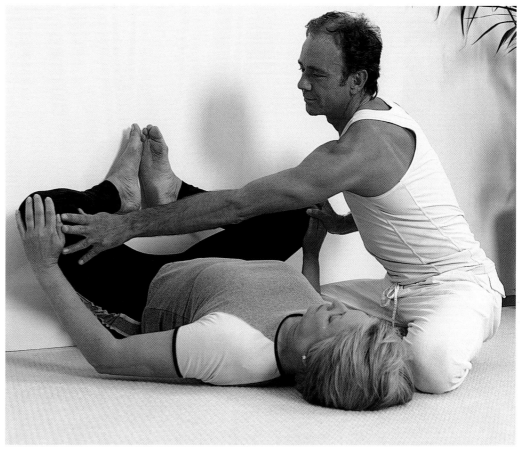

6 With arms wide open, bend the knees and draw the feet on to the soles. Have the feet hip-width apart and about 18 in. (45 cm) from the buttocks. **Exhaling,** lower the right knee to the left foot and contract the right buttock muscles to open the hip. Root the shoulders and arms to the floor to provide stability. Expand the chest. The dynamic of this posture is most noticeable in the hips and the rotation of the abdominal organs. Inhale, raise the right leg, and repeat to the other side. Alternate from side to side, increasing the extension and release with each repetition. Exhaling, stretch the body flat.

This completes one cycle of Supine sequence III.

By giving the breath primacy,

musculo-skeletal alignment is

clarified by necessity.

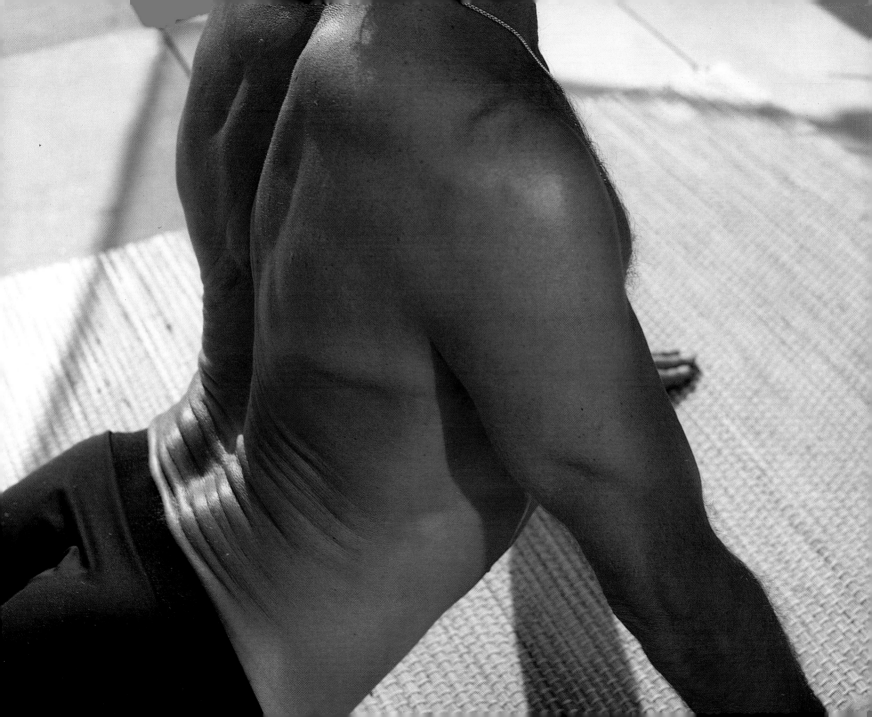

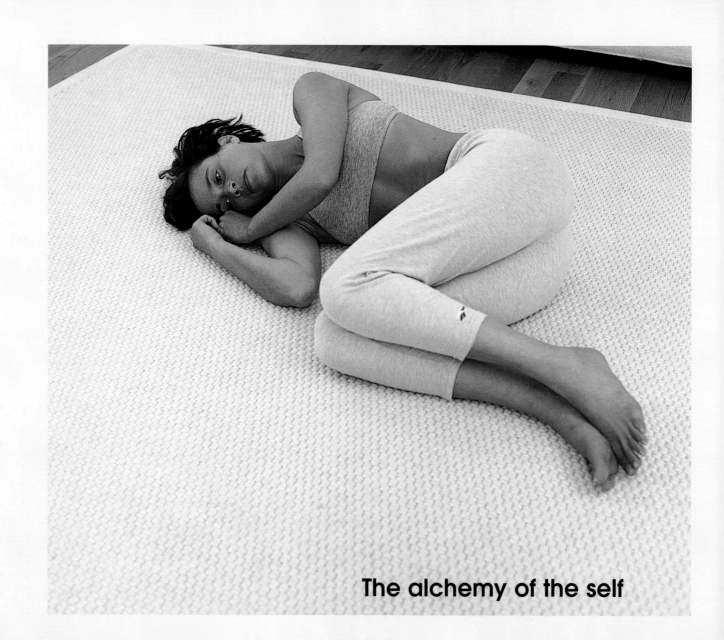

Relaxation

The alchemy of the self

During the activity of the postures, our obvious, or gross, form demands attention. The postures are designed to harness the mind and are literally a physical mandala. One of the advantages delivered by the practice of the postures is that they open the pathways of energy, stimulating the flow of vital energy throughout the body. This stimulation produces subtle vibrations and delicate sensations, which become the focus of attention in the practice of relaxation.

Just as expansion is countered by contraction, so activity must be balanced by passivity. The practice of relaxation is therefore an integral and important facet of the whole process of unification, it is a scientific art and not an opportunity for a short nap or a state of vacant unconsciousness. Drawing the mind deep into the body to explore and make contact with the subtle sensations of energy flow has the effect of opening the inner organs of perception and at the same time awakening the innate intelligence of the body. This is where the true nature of yoga or unity begins to reveal itself. As all of the bio-energy systems of the body slow down and assume a condition of repose, so does the thinking process.

* The body—our form—softens,
* the breathing process dissolves,
* and the mind expands and opens.

Each of the component parts of the tri-unity of our being—the body, spirit, and mind—are thus treated and brought to a state of equality and integral harmony.

The Sanskrit word for the conscious practice of relaxation is *Savasana*. This loosely translates as the "corpse" pose, referring to the fact that our usual conception of our bodies dies in relaxation and the true nature of form as being countless molecules and atoms vibrating freely in space is revealed. As the inner eye of intelligence further opens, our awareness of ourselves as a vibrant, essentially formless field of pure energy, the release of deeply held, residual tension, and the absorption of fresh vital energy is promoted. The structural reorganization and realignment of the body initiated by the information supplied by the postures can now be thoroughly digested. This transmission of understanding can only take place through the direct and conscious application of awareness—and awareness necessitates the absence of commentary, it is the silent impersonal witness, which feels, but does not judge. This means that when relaxing you should not try to evaluate the sensations you feel, but simply watch, follow, and indulge them.

The technique employed to encourage and increase an ability to effect this process is as simple as it is profound. However, as already stated, it is an art and science, and therefore, as with any fine art or form of study, it requires precise, diligent, and regular practice.

The benefits of deep relaxation

As the mind gains the ability to notice and stay fixed upon the subtle interplay of energy in the body, it also develops the power to influence and direct this essential, vital life-stream intelligently and purposefully. The soles of the feet produce one of the most obvious examples of our ability to increase the flow and dissolution of negative energy. Simply by maintaining inner awareness, the soles of the feet begin to discharge the effects of the gravitational pull and the weight of the body, which is borne by the feet throughout our waking life. Holding the inner gaze on the soles of the feet vastly increases the stream of negative energy out of the feet. The longer attention is given to this feeling, the greater the release of tension. This principle is true

Reaching a true state of relaxation

Although relaxation is practiced lying down flat on the floor, it is a posture first and foremost. Just as with any posture, pay attention to the correct alignment of the body. This is particularly important as you are creating a template or mold, which in time is imprinted upon the body/mind and therefore encourages proper structural alignment. The deliberate placement of the body also establishes the quality of mind necessary to derive the maximum benefits of practice.

• Make sure the spine feels centered and the back of the trunk is spread evenly on the floor.

• Lengthen the trunk and spine as you take the back of the head from the shoulders.

• Stretch the legs out of the hips, opening the lower back. This action ensures the spine is opened vertebra by vertebra, which in turn releases and broadens the shoulders.

• Stretch the arms out at the sides of the body and push the palms of the hands into the floor. Take a deep in-breath and at the same time squeeze together the feet and legs and press the whole body into the ground.

• The following exhalation is quite short but obvious, it indicates the release of exertion and establishes repose. During this release of the breath, the feet fall away from each other and the hands turn so the palms face the sky.

• Replace deep resonant breathing with sensitive, subtle, and automatic breath.

• It is still just as important to pay attention to the quality of each breath, but you need no longer exert any influence or control. Simply watch as the mechanics of the respiratory system dissolve until the impact of the breath becomes virtually imperceptible.

• Direct the initial point of focus to the heaviness of the back of the body and the relinquishment of the body's weight to the gravity of the earth. This instigates the dissolution of tension and the absorption of negative, stale energy into the ground.

• Once the process of dissolution has begun, bring awareness to the back of the eyes.

• Soften the eyeballs and look down toward the tip of the nose.

• Feel the coolness and sensitivity of the in-breath at the back of the eyes and let it suffuse into the sinus chambers and skull.

• Lighten and lift the forehead and let the two hemispheres of the brain separate and open. The back of the brain contracts and seems heavy, and as a direct result of the softening of brain tissue, the muscles of the face release and an environment of introspective awareness is established.

• From here it is simply a matter of attending to the various aspects of the body with an increasing sense of attention to detail. Attending to the details provides the means to access the essence of the whole; conversely, externally viewing the whole only reveals the obvious and the mundane.

and applicable to every facet of the body, and this is how the practice continues.

From the feet, allow the mind's eye to move slowly up, sequentially through the body, deepening contact and intimacy. Give special attention to the softness and openness of the solar plexus and the release of the diaphragm wall, as this area houses our emotional brain, and freedom here liberates the heart muscle. There is a substantial and noticeable increase in energy distribution as the heart is free to expand and contract without any impedance. As all of the other bio-energy systems slip into a state of suspended animation, fresh, highly oxygenated blood circulates evenly and effectively and the whole body/mind is bathed in the golden glow of its own awareness.

Reawaken the body slowly

Due to the direct and powerful impact of this process upon the nervous system, it is imperative that the subsequent arousal of the body/mind is done with the utmost care and attention.

* Begin stirring the body/mind by moving just one finger or toe. No matter how delicate or sensitive, this slight action shatters the equilibrium and former expansive awareness previously established. It is like a thunderclap on a still moonlit night that echoes throughout the whole body/mind.

* Realizing the profound effect that even the most delicate movement has upon the body/mind, the following movements are made with the same introspective awareness and are gradually increased in range and scope.

* Moving from the fingers and toes, the peripheral areas of the body are awakened first.

* The ankles and wrists are rotated, which gently stimulates the legs, arms, and spine and as muscle, bone, ligament, and tendon resume their function, the rest of the body begins to open and express itself.

Renewing your connection with daily life

This reawakening of the body is such a wonderful opportunity to enjoy the results of the practice. The body feels lithe, articulate, and supple. The mind feels open, unhurried, and refreshed. A natural ease and simple joy of being manifests, which is heightened as the whole body is animated by the kind of deep and rejuvenatory stretch made following a short nap after a leisurely Sunday lunch.

Rolling and resting on the right-hand side of the body for a minute or two ensures that pressure is not placed upon the heart wall and also gently stimulates the muscles, organs, and nerves of the body without coercion. The trick now is to appreciate and integrate this quiescence and subtle awareness into everyday life. The practice of relaxation is a technique that must be translated into everyday life if it is to have any true benefit. The practice is not a device that enables us to escape from reality. It is, indeed, a fine and incisive tool, which cuts through the external layers of form and reveals the essence of being. This quality of being is omnipresent; it is always there—all you have to do is to take the time to look. These relaxation postures will help you in your search.

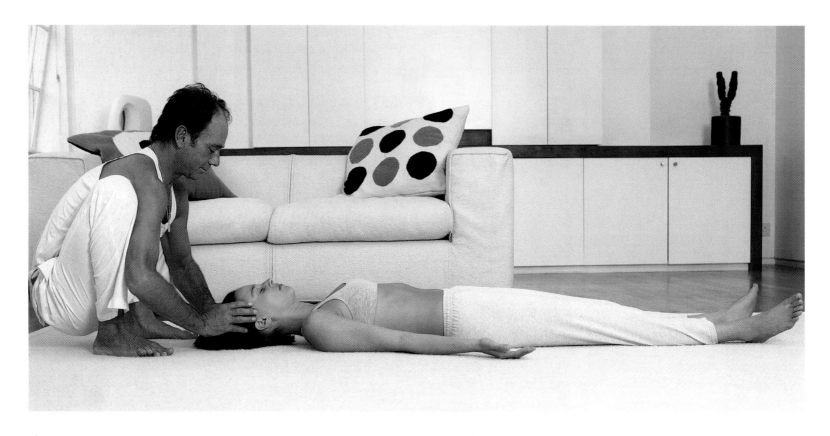

▲ PURE AND SIMPLE

• NEVER CASUALLY FLOP ON TO THE FLOOR AFTER PRACTICE.

• ALWAYS CHECK CAREFULLY THAT THE WHOLE BODY, FROM THE CROWN OF THE HEAD TO THE TIPS OF THE TOES, IS LENGTHENED AND EVENLY SPREAD.

PURE AND SIMPLE ▶

• IF ANY DISCOMFORT IS FELT IN THE LOWER BACK, IT IS PERFECTLY ACCEPTABLE TO LIE WITH THE KNEES BENT, RESTING AGAINST EACH OTHER. SPEND TIME FOCUSING ON ANY RESIDUAL TENSION.

• NOTICE HOW THIS PROMOTES DISSOLUTION AND RELIEVES STRAIN. THE LEGS SHOULD BE STRAIGHTENED OUT ONCE THE DISCOMFORT HAS EASED.

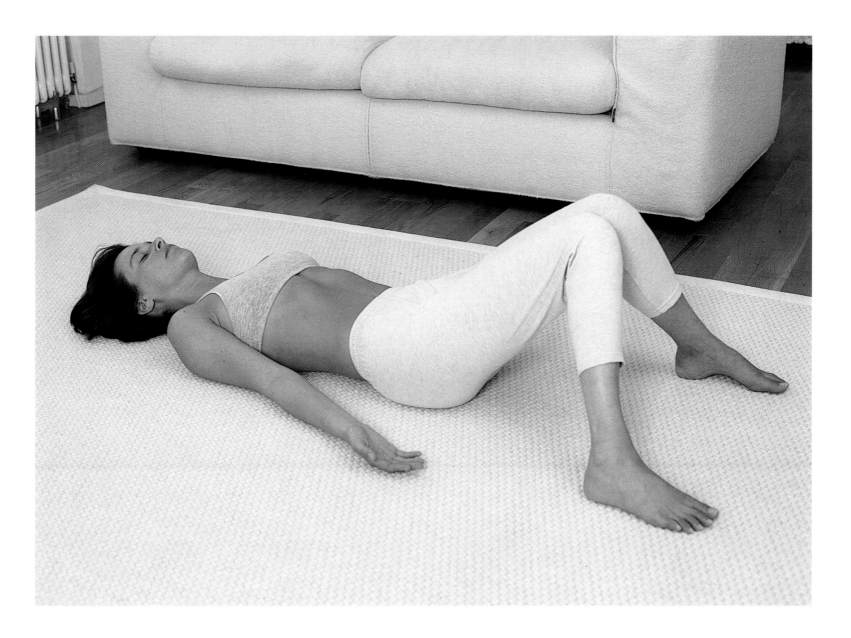

Awareness necessitates the absence of commentary. It is the silent impersonal witness, which feels but does not judge.

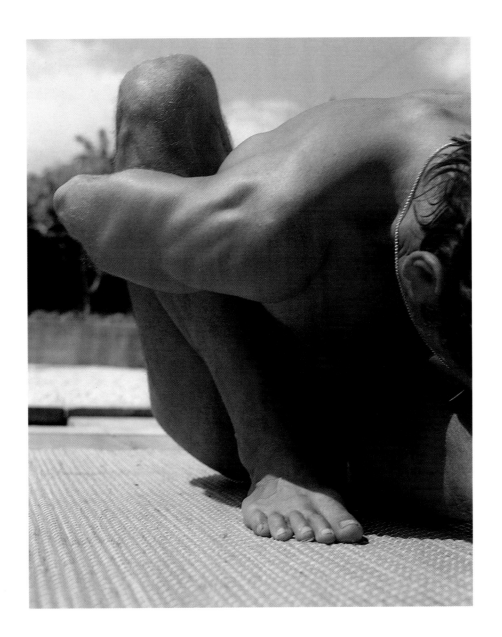

Meditation

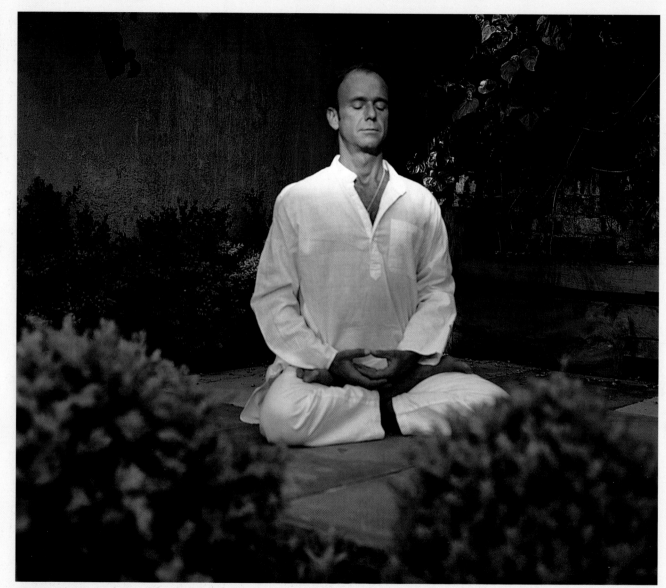

Harvest moon

There is nothing more valuable than a peaceful mind. If our mind is turbulent and unsettled, it discolors our lives. No matter how idyllic our surroundings, no matter how bright the sun shines, how sweetly the birds sing, or how fit and healthy we appear, if our minds are agitated, we will be blind to the magic that is our lives. Sitting meditation is the practice that enables us to restore balance and order to the fluctuations of the mind. It provides us with the skillful means to embrace life in all its forms and to take personal responsibility for the quality of mind we bring to any particular situation, circumstance, or event.

From an early age, we are taught that we are all born with free will; our birthright is "choice." But we cannot choose to be a glamor model if we don't have the looks; we cannot be a great artist if we do not have the skill; we cannot choose our parents, our children, our race, or our color. In fact, we have very little choice about anything in absolute terms.

So what is it that we can choose? The only real and effective choice we have is the color of mind that we bring to any and every given situation we meet. The whole ambience of our actual state is governed by the quality and receptivity of our mind. The capacity of our mind to receive is directly linked to the degree and the level of awareness of ourselves as individuals living in a world of independent interdependence. Awareness is the master key that unlocks the heavy, solid casket that contains all our worst fears, loathing, insecurities, and self-importance. In this respect, meditation is an exercise in multidimensional awareness.

It is through this practice that the other disciplines gain strength and fulfill their purpose and not the other way around. We are too often seduced by conventional ideas of fitness, and the increase in energy and vitality offered by the practice of the postures. The postures are such obvious devices and tempt us with offers of svelte waistlines, great strength, stamina, and, of course, flexibility that we can, just about, make time for them with a quick relaxation thrown in at the end. However, the purpose of the postures is not to ensure or promote weight reduction or to manufacture extraordinary contortions for the amusement of our friends. Their true purpose and greatness is that they introduce the component parts of our being to each other. The body is activated, energized, and revealed to the mind during the activity of the postures. In relaxation, energy and mind saturate the body and in the practice of meditation, body, energy, and mind galvanize, become one.

The direct involvement of each of the aspects of our being has the effect of opening our inner organs of perception, which allows us to investigate and explore the various facets of our psycho-physiological make-up. Our fears, loathings, repressions, preferences, and prejudices, together with our strengths and finer qualities, are all revealed under the cool light of an open, expansive mind. It is from this impassive, tranquil condition that integration is developed and meaningful, transformative insights appear.

- Wisdom is the skillful use of the energy that is our life form.
- Wisdom describes the ability to act appropriately, regardless of circumstance.
- The wise are just as likely to encounter difficulty as anyone else; floods, natural disasters, life, and death are not dismissed by wisdom, rather, difficulties and problems are embraced and dealt with expediently and efficiently, regardless of personal preference or cost.
- Wisdom grows from panoramic awareness, which in turn is developed through deep self-examination and introspection.

The benefits of meditation

In sitting meditation, the mind turns inward and investigates its environment, its habitual patterns of action, its resistances and desires, and gradually sees that they are ultimately insubstantial. The direct, experiential witnessing of the transience of all things disempowers fears, loathing, and resistance and generates a mind that is then free, open, and revealing. We cannot ever be totally free from the inconveniences of life or successfully turn ourselves into a perfect picture of how we should be. But we can do something, we can look and see and feel who and what we actually are beyond any preconceived notions, ideals, and principles of how we should behave.

I remember early on in my Zen practice my teacher, Genpo Merzel Roshi, telling me that if I had come to this practice to become a better person, I would be wasting my time and would only be disappointed. I didn't realize quite what he meant at the time, and it wasn't until much later that the significance of his statement dawned upon me. I had, without realizing it, been trying to whitewash my former life, almost attempting to bleach away any stain or seeming imperfection. The practice is not one of abstinence or denial. In total contrast, it is a means to proper, relaxed being. This is a deep sense of inner relaxation with our composite selves in the diversity of our circumstances. We cannot get rid of the sinner; we can only get rid of the judge.

The judgemental mind sees everything from a narrow perspective, right and wrong, good and bad, should and should not, and even fat-thin, pretty-ugly, nice and nasty. This removes us from the underlying reality of our lives and limits our life to one of mere conformity. Reality does not give a hoot whether you are tall or short; it makes no comment and is beyond the confines of preference. Wishing things to be other than they are removes us from the great reality and transfers us to the realms of misery and self-centeredness.

Taking the time to sit and bear witness to our own absolute reality establishes a direct and confident connection with life itself. Self-importance is replaced with self-confidence, and this in turn unleashes any aspects previously considered negative and directs their power to the pure and simple art of being.

In meditation, the quality of mind established by the process of relaxation is allied with the activity and understanding of the body, developed through the practice of the postures and awareness of the breath. This balance creates an atmosphere of dignity and inner composure as harmony between tension and relaxation brings about the right tension.

• Use the inner eye of intelligence to maintain a subtle but firm grip on the body to ensure the posture does not slacken.
• Keep the body alive and the mind alert and attentive; the feeling this produces is one of dynamic stillness.

When the inner eye and the inner ear open, inner quiet is revealed. Silence is not the goal, however; it is simply the means by which incisive, tender intimacy is developed. This state of consciousness is not vacant or empty. In fact, it reveals an acute awareness of plenitude. It is full, active, expressive, and deep.

Preparing for meditation

The first hurdle you face is not in silencing the mind or curtailing the inner dialogue, it is in maintaining perfection of the posture. Choose a place that is quiet, clean, and tidy for practice as the simpler and more appealing the environment the easier it will be to relax. The full Lotus posture is the best position to adopt for sitting meditation as it provides the perfect base for the spine to lift and extend up out of the pelvic girdle.

- Take the left leg and bend it at the knee.
- Draw the left foot high up and on to the right thigh. The sole of the foot should face the sky with the heel close to the navel.
- Next, bend the right leg and take the right foot over the left shin and up to the root of the left thigh so both heels are close to each other with the feet balanced and even.

Depending upon your degree of flexibility and length of practice, this position can be quite intense and demands a great deal of practice before it becomes comfortable. It is therefore not recommended for beginners. There are alternatives that are more accommodating and can be used by most people without discomfort.

- Sit astride two or three cushions, with the knees wide and the bridges of the feet flat on the floor.
- Make sure that you do not sink into the cushions and that they offer firm support.
- Ensure that the cushions provide enough height to allow the pelvis to tilt forward and consequently for the spine to draw in.

Alternatively, adopt the basic crossed-legs position where the feet and legs are forward and close together. In this position, a single cushion is generally used, as it offers stability.

- All of the principles established concerning the accurate alignment of the body in the postures are obviously applicable in this simple seat for meditation.
- The bridges of the feet roll down to the floor with one heel close to the pubis and the other directly in front of the first.
- Try to keep the center of both heels in line and vertical. Placing the feet in this way rotates the thighbones, which is the essential action necessary to allow the spine to draw in and lift up.

Whichever form you choose, it is essential that the spine lifts up straight and strong, the arms are a little open, and the hands come together to produce a careful and delicate gesture called the universal mudra, or seal.

- Place the right hand on top of the left so that the middle joints of the knuckles come together and the tips of the thumbs lightly touch so the shape the hands describe is a perfect oval.
- Lift up the chest so the diaphragm is soft and open, and encourage the crown of the head to aspire to reach the sky.
- With the chin parallel to the floor, curl back the tongue and press the tip against the front of the roof of the palate. This detail retards the flow of saliva and also has a direct influence upon the brain, as a small plexus of nerves are located at this point.
- The application of a little pressure here slows down brain patterns, and therefore the thinking process.

By adopting this systematic and attentive approach to sitting meditation, you induce an atmosphere that promotes a calm and contemplative condition.

Meditating through breathing

The basic technique and foundation of all meditative practices is to simply count each breath. This is a device that anchors and trains the mind to stay present and attendant simultaneously. It also has the benefit of increasing intimacy and awareness of our breath and its direct relationship with the thinking process, and also reveals the transient nature of all things. Gradually you will notice that without trying, your breath has become finer, more delicate, and as a direct result the whole ambience of your being has also become softer, more receptive, and content. Therefore, it is important to keep the breath natural, without influence or support other than a slight tensing of the abdominal muscles at the end of each out-breath. This may seem to be a very easy exercise, but such is the strong pull of the discursive mind that it proves to be quite tricky. In fact, some people find they can count each breath and indulge the inner dialogue at the same time. This is neither the practice nor the way to progress. Determine to apply yourself wholeheartedly to the task and register each time that thinking overrides counting.

• Sitting up straight and strong, with the eyes directed toward the floor in a soft misty gaze, breathe out gently but quite deeply.

• As the following inhalation seeps into the chambers of the upper nasal cavities, count one.

• On the out-breath, count two and so on until a count of ten has been reached.

• Then start again, repeating the process for a period of 10 to 20 minutes to begin with.

• Watch carefully that stray thoughts do not develop into conversations, as the practice is to pay attention to the discipline of counting and the maintenance of the form. Once the technique has been mastered, counting can be dispensed with, and pure awareness of the breath is developed instead.

Meditating through visualization

The second technique uses the practice of visualization as a means to direct the mind. This often tends to be a more accessible means of meditation for some, as there is a certain personal connection. It is just as difficult to master as counting the breath, as we can become easily drawn into the realms of the past, future, and fantasy. Once again, the posture is of utmost importance, the only difference between the former posture and this method is that the eyes are closed; all of the other instructions equally apply.

• Breathing out, draw the inner gaze to the tip of the nose and visualize the person closest to you. Usually this is your partner, parent, or child. Encourage their image to appear in the solar plexus—the emotional heart-center—for just enough time to send the feeling of love and affection to them.

• Continue by moving to the next person you feel a strong emotional bond with. Once you have visualized all your family, friends, neighbors, and fellow workers expand the range by introducing people who serve you in shops, restaurants, and bars; indeed, anyone with whom you have regular contact.

• Try not to fall into the trap of dwelling upon any one person as this will only lead down the road of illusion and away from the single-minded path of concentrated awareness.

• As this is a practice that develops universal compassion and devotion, make sure you give the same degree of love and affection to the people who annoy and irritate you as you do to those closest to you.

• Expand the mind-field to include everyone who lives in the same street as you and then out further to the neighborhood, town, or city. Open to the country you live in, offering every inhabitant the same quality of mind, and do not stop until the whole world has been embraced by the heart-mind.

The combined power of all of these techniques is tremendous, and the rewards are felt not just by the practitioner but also by everyone they touch and meet. The equanimity and peace we find within ourselves cannot be enjoyed in isolation. Their quality is reflected in every aspect of our being.

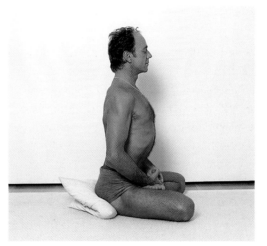 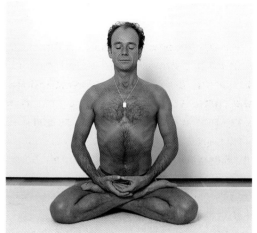

Patience, perseverance, and frequency are the qualities necessary to master the full Lotus posture. Take great care in bending the knees and placing the feet on the soft flesh of the thighs, making sure the knee joints are not displaced or misaligned in the process. Sitting on the front third of the cushion allows the pelvis to tilt forward and the trunk and spine to lift up. This is one of the most noble and satisfying of all the yoga postures. It opens the hips, makes the leg muscles soft and flexible, and delivers a sense of calm authority and self-composure.

Meditation is an exercise in multidimensional awareness.

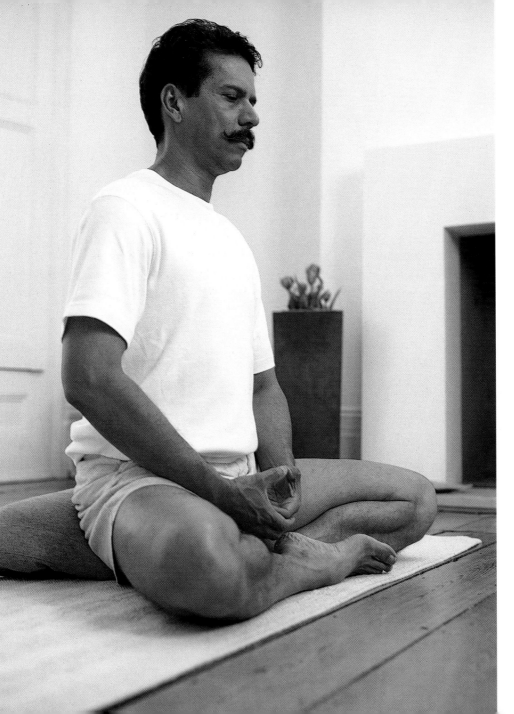

PURE AND SIMPLE

• SIT ON THE FRONT THIRD OF THE
CUSHION WITH BOTH KNEES ON THE
FLOOR, AS THIS PROVIDES THE
NECESSARY TILT OF THE PELVIS, WHICH
ALLOWS THE SPINE TO LIFT.

• TUCK THE HEAD AND CHIN BACK JUST
A LITTLE TO ENCOURAGE THE OPENING
OF THE CHEST AND SOLAR PLEXUS.

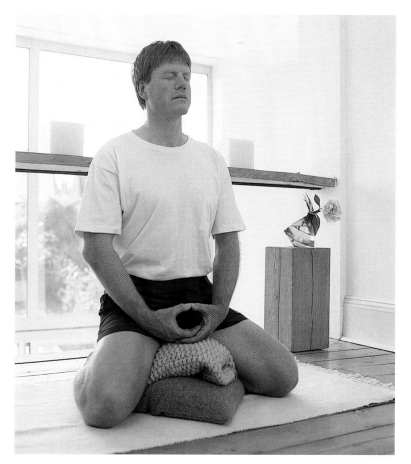

PURE AND SIMPLE

• ADJUST THE HEIGHT OF THE CUSHIONS TO SUIT YOUR NEEDS, MAKING SURE THEY PROVIDE SUFFICIENT SUPPORT AND COMFORT.

• ALTHOUGH THIS POSTURE IS THE EASIEST TO MAINTAIN, IT ALSO PRODUCES THE MOST IMMEDIATE DISCOMFORT UPON RELEASE. THEREFORE, IT IS WISE TO GENTLY AND SENSITIVELY STRETCH THE LEGS AFTER MEDITATING IN THIS POSTURE.

• OVER TIME, THE SENSATIONS IN THE LEGS ARE GRADUALLY EASED AS THE LEG MUSCLES SOFTEN AND THE MIND CEASES TO REACT.

The body is activated, energized, and revealed to the mind during

the activity of the postures. In relaxation, energy and mind saturate

the body and in the practice of meditation, body, energy, and mind

galvanize, becoming one.

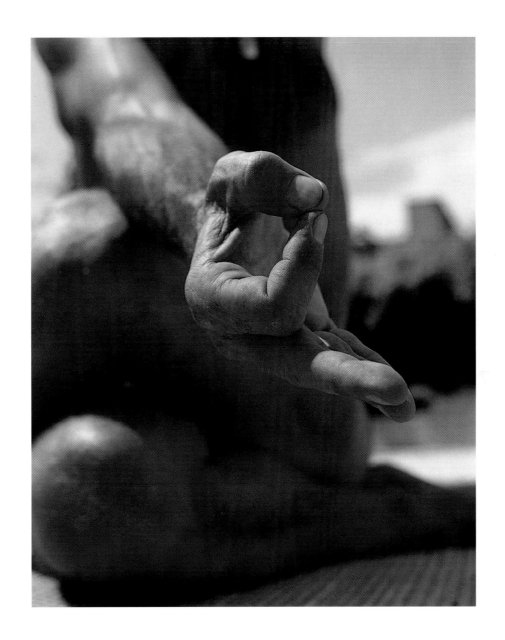

Creating your own sequences

The following sequences are designed to further and encourage personal practice. They are stuctured by periods of time and are simply a guide to expanding and developing practice. As experience and understanding grow, they can be modified and adapted to suit individual needs and circumstance.

1 15–20 minutes, morning

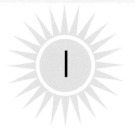

Sun sequence I,
as seen on page 20

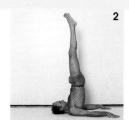 1
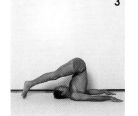 2
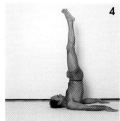 3
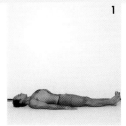 4
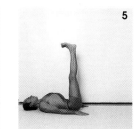 5

Inverted sequence I,
as seen on page 88

2 15–20 minutes, morning

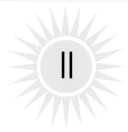

Sun sequence II,
as seen on page 26

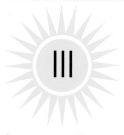

Sun sequence III,
as seen on page 32

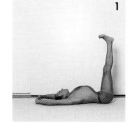 1
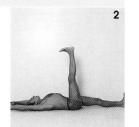 2
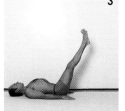 3
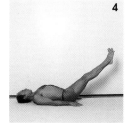 4

Supine sequence I,
as seen on page 110

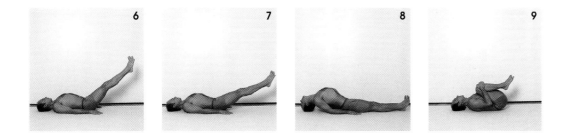

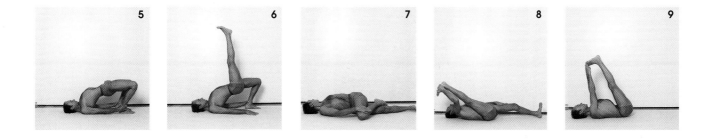

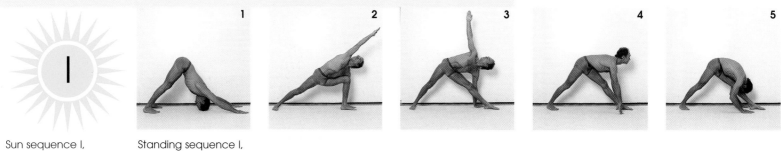

Sun sequence I,
as seen on page 20

Standing sequence I,
as seen on page 44

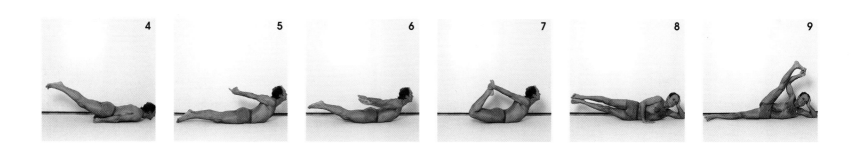

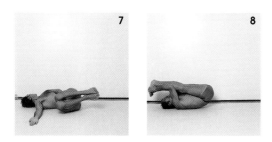

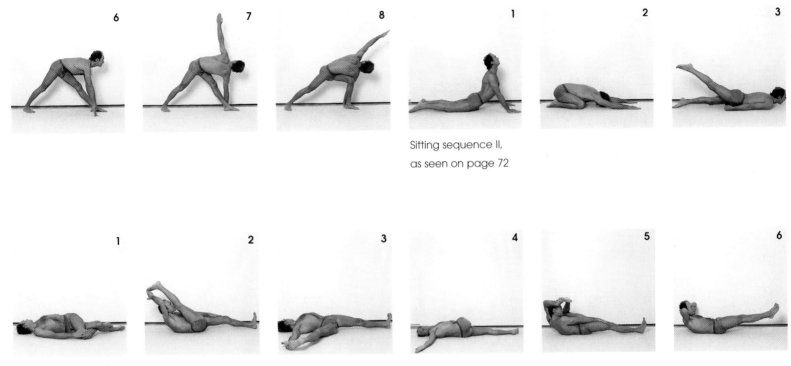

Sitting sequence II,
as seen on page 72

Supine sequence II,
as seen on page 116

4 40–60 minutes, morning

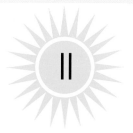

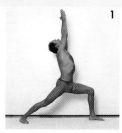
1

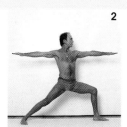
2

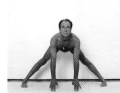
3

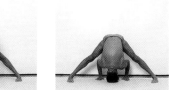
4

5

Sun sequence II,
as seen on page 26

Standing sequence II,
as seen on page 50

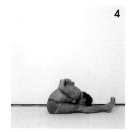
4

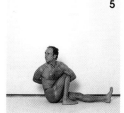
5

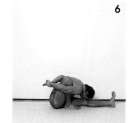
6

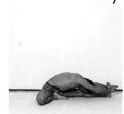
7

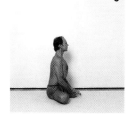
8

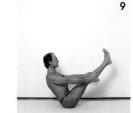
9

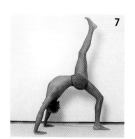
7

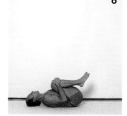
8

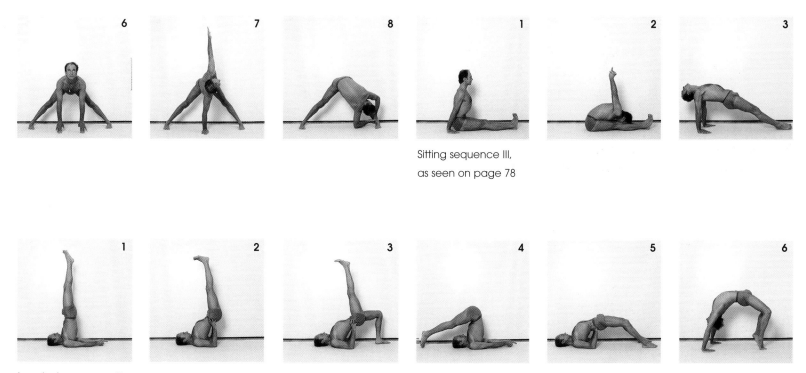

Sitting sequence III,
as seen on page 78

Inverted sequence III,
as seen on page 100

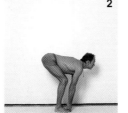 1

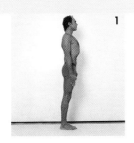 2

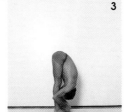 3

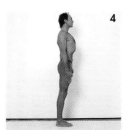 4

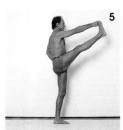 5

Sun sequence I,
as seen on page 20

Standing sequence III,
as seen on page 56

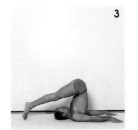 3

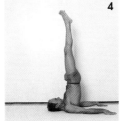 4

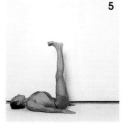 5

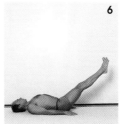 6

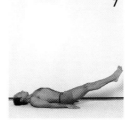 7

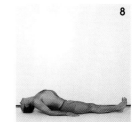 8

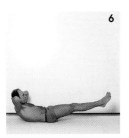 6

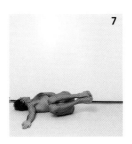 7

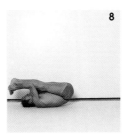 8

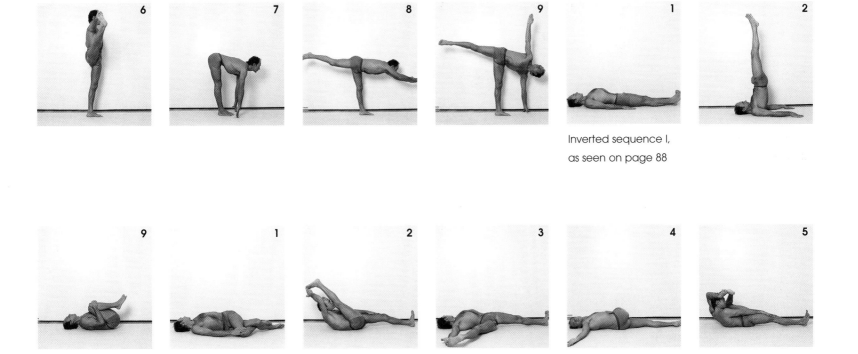

Inverted sequence I,
as seen on page 88

Supine sequence II,
as seen on page 116

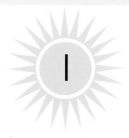

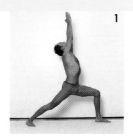

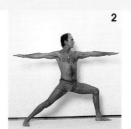

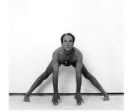

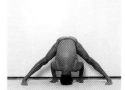

Sun sequence I,
as seen on page 20

Standing sequence II,
as seen on page 50

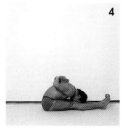

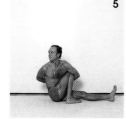

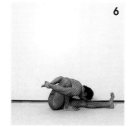

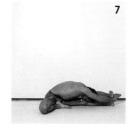

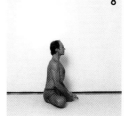

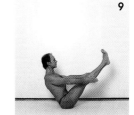

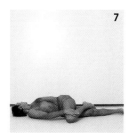

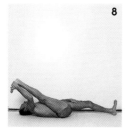

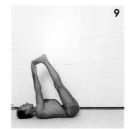

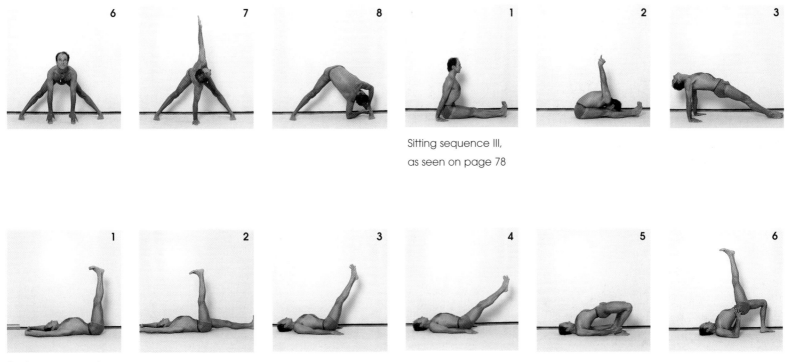

Sitting sequence III,
as seen on page 78

Supine sequence I,
as seen on page 110

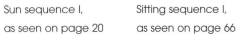

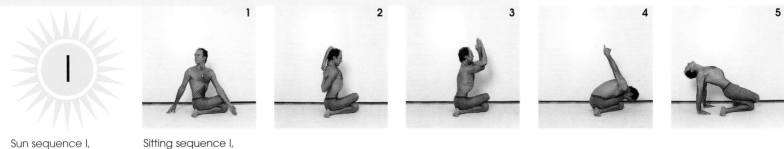

Sun sequence I,
as seen on page 20

Sitting sequence I,
as seen on page 66

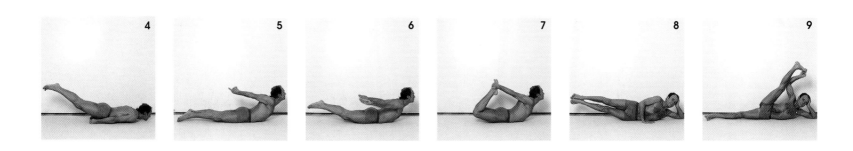

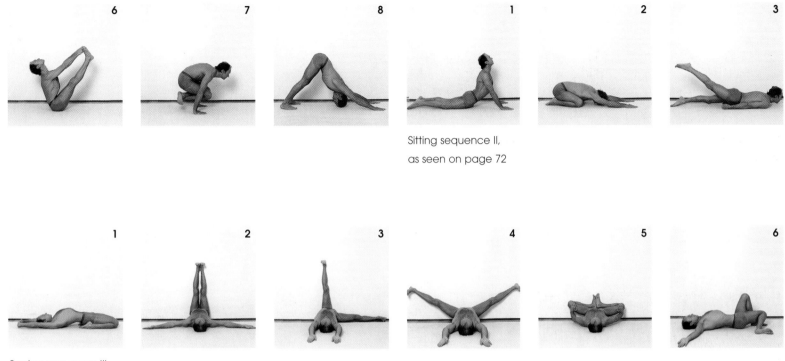

Sitting sequence II,
as seen on page 72

Supine sequence III,
as seen on page 122

Author's acknowledgments

I would like to take this opportunity to offer my deepest gratitude to all of the students I have met over the course of my teaching. I have learned so much from you all. A special mention must be given for their kindness, generosity, and support to:

Sir David, Sir Frederick, and Lady Berkeley, Margaret Castleton, Suzy Chappell, Paul, Monique, and Etienne De Villiers, Amanda Eliasch, Francesca French, Julie Gadd, Daniella Gareh, Anne Gilding, Rita, Pia, and Arjun Gadkari, Geri Halliwell, Honey Luard, Emily Owen, Suzi Papallios, Jennifer Pettit, Jimmy Rogan, Tom Stephan, David Wilson, and Sam Taylor-Wood.

And also to Amanda Berkeley, Paul Brewer, Tracy Brower, Anita De Villiers, Emma Louise Field, and Vilas Gadkari for kindly allowing themselves to be photographed for this book. I would also like to thank them for their keenness and embodiment of practice.

To Lisa Gibbs whose love and care helped me through the project.

I should also like to thank everyone at Ebury Press for their help and guidance. In particular, Helen Lewis for her care and attention; Emma Callery for her insight, understanding, and great patience; and Denise Bates for providing me with such a wonderful opportunity.

Finally, I should like to offer my deep gratitude and love to Godfrey Devereaux and Genpo Merzel Roshi for their guidance, inspiration, and love.

I can never repay the debt I owe you all.

Thank you. Gassho.

Kisen

We hope you enjoyed this Hay House book. If you would like to receive a free catalog featuring additional Hay House books and products, or if you would like information about the Hay Foundation, please contact:

Hay House, Inc.
P.O. Box 5100
Carlsbad, CA 92018-5100

(760) 431-7695 or **(800) 654-5126**
(760) 431-6948 (fax) or **(800) 650-5115 (fax)**

Please visit the Hay House Website at:
www.hayhouse.com